50 Shades
of
Curious

Bo Blaze, PCC

Published by:

50 Shades of Curious
370 W. Pleasantview Ave #300
Hackensack, NJ 07601
info@50ShadesOfCurious.com

ISBN: 978-0-9885009-0-7
ISBN-10: 0988500906

Library of Congress Control Number: 2012951714

DISCLAIMER

The materials presented are for "Informational and Entertainment Purposes Only". The very nature of these activities dictates that there is inherent risk of personal injury while carrying them out. All BDSM activities involve a potential risk for serious injury and all activities are undertaken entirely at the readers own risk. Although we believe the information in this presentation to be accurate and timely, we make no warranty or guarantee concerning the accuracy or reliability of the content or other material which we may reference. This presentation is provided in an "as is" format without warranties of any kind, expressed or implied.

TES Creed ©1971 - 2012,
Used with permission
The Eulenspiegel Society/The TES Association

Author Photograph: LC Misfit Studios

DEDICATION

This book is dedicated to my
wife, partner, rock, bean, and hedly
Siouxsie Blaze

CONTENTS

DEDICATION iii

CONTENTS v

ACKNOWLEDGMENTS...1

FORWARD...3

INTRODUCTION..7

GETTING STARTED 11

COMMUNICATION 23

CONSENT..49

RELATIONSHIPS...61

YOUR IDENTITY 81

PAIN & PUNISHMENT.....................................109

TOYS & ACTIVITIES...119

THE MENTAL SIDE 141

SAFETY 155

READING LIST 181

BO'ISMS...189

ABOUT THE AUTHOR...191

INDEX...192

ACKNOWLEDGMENTS

I first want to thank my wife, Siouxsie, and my *girls*, Anna and Dee. You put up with me, you take care of me, you love me. No one could ask for more loyal, loving souls to share my life with.

I also need to thank both my *Sovereign House* and bio families for all their support and love over the years.

So many people have taught me so much over the years I don't know where to start. But thank you to every friend, educator, scene and every person who has ever given me the gift of knowledge.

There have been a few people that I consider special mentors and friends along my journey. Some I have spent many hours with and others much less, but they have all influenced me profoundly, just the same: Philip Miller, Molly Devon, Lolita Wolf, Master Taino, Flagg, Pat Bond, Jeff R, Uncle Mike, Brian Drago, Colin Regina, Phil Pfisterer, Vance Aun, Tim Vasile, Ben Malin, Peter & Denise Blasevick, Laine Campbell Walter Gemeinhardt , Fred Azizaj, James Campion Joe Luddy, Tom Scarsone

And those that have guided me through their words and actions: J. Krishnamurti, Bill Hicks, Tim Ferriss

Many thanks to Karen Walk for her excellent transcription work, Nimmy Philip for his indispensable editing, and Lauren for her proofreading.

ACKNOWLEDGMENTS

FORWARD

During our life journeys, we come across very unique individuals who we connect with. Sometimes, we do not even know why or where the connections come from.

That was how it was many years ago when I met Bo Blaze. Our paths crossed and the mutual respect and admiration was almost instantaneous. It seemed at that time that Bo and I did not have much in common. To start, he was a straight kinky guy and I was a gay leatherman. It happens that one of his partners was a member of the Defenders Leather Levi Club in New York while I was a member of the Washington DC chapter, and that facilitated us getting to know each other a bit more.

At that time, back in the mid-nineties, I was very safe in my gay box, and did not know many straight kinky folks. I remember noticing that the fact that I was gay did not have any effect on Bo. He was, and still is, his own man, always smiling and friendly.

Through the years, we kept seeing each other at events, and developed a great friendship. I soon discovered that we actually do have many things in common. To start, he is very passionate about flogging, and even owns a business that sells them. And I live to flog. That mutual passion for flogging was cemented when he invited me to be part of his DVD *The Details of Flogging*, which allowed me to introduce my cathartic flogging experience to a whole new market. It also allowed me to visit him at his home where we did the filming and got to spend some quality time in his New Jersey coastal town on a rainy autumn evening.

Bo and I also share our visions for a leather family. We both have derived a great deal of satisfaction from forming multiple relationships with individuals who may not be biological family, but have become members of our true family, just the same.

Probably most importantly, we both share another passion. We both spend a great deal of our life journeys helping the next generation of kinky folks, the novices or "newbies" who come into our leather communities. With the arrival of the Internet in the last quarter century, the leather, BDSM, fetish, and power exchange dynamics have flourished, particularly among the younger crowd, whose members are freer to explore their sexuality in less traditional ways.

These young folks, the new generation that is coming up and discovering our world, need the guidance and mentoring of more experienced kinky folks. Not everyone has the patience, the desire, the wisdom and the passion to teach and mentor new folks. It requires people with a deep commitment to assisting the inexperienced and education.

Bo Blaze is one of those folks. Like myself, he has that passion to reach out, help, mentor, guide, assist, teach and develop young people with an interest in BDSM and power exchange relationships. For years, he has been particularly dedicated to reaching out to the novices in the New York and New Jersey area. Our common view of our responsibility toward our community and the younger generation has allowed our

4

friendship and our mutual respect to grow deeper year after year.

Writing a book is no easy task. It takes time and dedication. With this effort, Bo has gone one step further to provide the new generation with an important tool to learn our craft. I hope that it serves its purpose and that many young folks can take advantage of the information that Bo provides here.

Master Taíno
2011 Pantheon of Leather Man of the Year

INTRODUCTION

As a PCC-certified "alternative" life coach, I specialize in working with alternative sexual relationships and non-traditional lifestyles, specifically, kink, lifestyle BDSM, ethical non-monogamy (polyamory), the fetish world and LGBT issues.

I've taught and lectured all over the country at hundreds of universities, conferences, and various alternative events. I have helped thousands of people learn to practice safe, sane and consensual (SSC) BDSM over the last 10 years as the Novice Group facilitator for The Eulenspiegel Society (TES) in NYC. TES is the oldest and largest BDSM support and education group in the country. I was also recently honored to receive The Pantheon of Leather President's award for my many years of work in our community.

So it's no wonder that many of my friends, and possibly you, the reader, may wonder why after years of working within these various real worlds I'd choose to name my book and entire educational system as an homage to a romance novel and one of the most polarizing books in the history of BDSM?

To answer that question properly, we must go back to the year 1969. On June 28th, 1969, at the Stonewall Inn in Greenwich Village, NYC, a group of gay customers took a stand against police harassment and the Stonewall Riots began. These riots are now largely regarded as the catalyst for the LGBT civil rights movement in the United States. It is generally looked at as "the moment that changed everything".

The riots themselves were not the reason that things changed, but they were a moment in time that we can point to when the bubble burst; It was a tipping point, when the publicity generated from an event brought mass attention to something long ignored that was on the edge of change.

The publishing of *Fifty Shades of Grey* is not the dawning of a literary masterpiece, a factually correct overview of how to do BDSM or a book that will likely be remembered any more than the drink menu and decor of the Stonewall Inn back in 1969. Like it or not, however, it's an important moment in history.

The USA Today has reported that *Fifty Shades of Grey* has sold over 32 million copies as of July 2012. It's now the biggest selling book of all time in the UK and the biggest selling book on the Kindle platform in the U.S. as well. When you look at how women are treating E.L.James, the writer of the book, you'd almost think she was the second coming of the Beatles. This kind of passion and sales success does not happen solely because of the content of a book, let alone one known as a "trashy romance novel".

No, this is a shift in culture! This is millions of women reclaiming their right to be whoever and whatever they want to be in the bedroom, regardless of their politics.

These are every day women from all walks of life, overwhelmingly voting YES on the "kinky sex referendum", saying: "we like a little spanking and hair pulling...what's wrong with that?" Most importantly, people are looking around at the crazy success of this book and realizing, evidently, A WHOLE LOT OF US have these interests, urges and fantasies.

And certainly NOT just dominant male/submissive female fantasies, but every combination and flavor that one can think of. These fetishes and predilections that we call BDSM are not about abuse; rather, they are about consensual intimacy in the bedroom.

For years, sex-positive feminists have embraced BDSM and opposed legal or social efforts to control any type of sexual activity between consenting adults. Now, without a bottle thrown or even a harsh word uttered, millions of women around the world have joined them and initiated a bloodless coup, inspired, by of all things, a romance novel.

I believe this is part of a bigger picture, however. Our world is changing for the better. We are evolving. People are starting to realize that our institutions and their dogmas are failing us because they have become irrelevant in our ever changing society.

We must move towards truth and away from fear.

As an alternative life coach, I want to help people live a more alternative life. To me, that simply means living a life where you are always growing, changing, and evolving. Where you question, think, and create. Where you refuse to settle for what you are told to do and instead follow a path to real fulfillment and enlightenment.

How you decide to manifest that is up to you, and kinky sex is just one small way you can begin to shake things up a bit in your life. Other ways you can shake up your life: refuse to settle for the norm; do something that you perhaps have always wanted to do, but were too embarrassed or scared to embrace; explore art, music, yoga, spirituality, service to your community or a new job doing what you really were meant to do!

When you stop growing, you start dying! Let's hope this is the year that it all changed. The year that a *silly* romance novel was the catalyst for an "earth shattering kaboom"! The year that we look back on and thank the universe that people are no longer persecuted, lose their children or shunned because of consensual acts in their bedrooms.

I recently sat down to lunch with my good friend Susan Wright, who is the founder of the *National Coalition of Sexual Freedom*. As we excitedly compared notes on the *50 shades of Grey* phenomenon, we were united in our belief that the reaction to this book could be a Stonewall of sorts for alternative sexuality. That this could open up the lines of communication and change everything. But to do that, it's going to take a lot of education and a lot of information.

Which brings me back to the name of this book, my website, and educational system. Simply put, I'm willing to be a whore to reach the masses. There are 32+ million people out there who have just read *Fifty Shades of Grey* and they have questions and need guidance as they begin their journey into BDSM and kinky sex. It's my mission to get them answers and do my best to keep them safe and well informed.

GETTING STARTED

You are about to begin a journey.

This journey may only take you as far as the bedroom door as you and your committed partner enjoy a hot new form of lovemaking. Or it might change your entire life and you'll find yourself in a strange, but wonderful, kinky world of people all interested in pushing the limits of their sexuality.

Whatever path you choose, there is something truly magical about the world of kinky sex and BDSM. It's very far away from what most people think it is. It's about growth and acceptance. It's about letting go of your fears and demons and not letting anyone tell you what SHOULD or should not make you sexually or mentally excited.

You'll find out things about what your partner(s) likes and take things that you like and you'll mix it all together and create something from nothing. A SCENE. It's like writing your own play or shooting your own movie, except you get to have an orgasm at the end if you want!

BDSM is a consensual activity. It is not abuse.

By definition, BDSM cannot exist without consent (meaning that everybody agrees). So, if you are doing something you consider to be BDSM, but all parties do not agree with what's going on, then what's happening is ABUSE, NOT BDSM.

Often, BDSM may include the illusion of non-consent, but at any point consent can be revoked and that is the difference between BDSM and abuse.

Two of my favorite mantras I preach to my novice group and coaching clients are:

There is no one right way to practice BDSM.

And

There are no rules in BDSM other than consent.

If somebody tells you something like

"You don't know what you are doing, You are no dominant!"

Or

"That's not how you are supposed to act when you're submissive!"

You should look them right in the eye, laugh at them, and walk away, because they do not have any right to tell you anything, and, frankly, they just don't *get it.*

Any person you would want to associate with in this world will defend your right to be exactly who you want to be. There is nothing to live up to since there are no hard and fast rules in BDSM, other than being consensual.

Just like in the vanilla world, the more obscure your interests, the harder it might be to find the partner you are looking for, but what you want is not *wrong*.

You'll certainly learn things or discover that you like the way this person does this and that person does that. But these are just models for you to work off of, ideas for you to take whatever you like and create your own *art*.

This is not a race, it's not about impressing other people, it's not about being the coolest or the best. This is about you and your partner(s) having a good time and getting your needs met. It's about CONNECTION with other human beings and honestly exploring your sexuality in whatever way you choose.

The 20-year scene veteran is no better than the person starting out for the first time. There is no amount of BDSM you should aspire to.

> *The person who is swinging from the chandeliers and using every kinky toy imaginable is no better than the person who just likes to get a little spanking before they have sex with their partner.*

As an alternative life coach, you should know that my motto is:

When you stop growing, you start dying.

And in order to keep growing we need to find various muses and activities to keep us from getting stagnant.

Mind/body and various creative endeavors, such as music, art, yoga, and things like that, do a great job of this. But one of my favorite mediums of choice would be alternative sexuality.

You might find it hard to believe that you can potentially grow as a person by spanking your partner, but by the time you're done reading this book I hope you understand what I mean when I say that you can. To aid that growth, I would also like to suggest you take heed of part two of my mantra, where I ask you to do your best to:

Let go of your fears

Seek truth

Find your integrity

Scene Speak

The following terms are used in the book, and it's best to understand them before you dive in. We'll be explaining some of these terms more in depth later in the book.

BDSM – Bondage and discipline (BD) and sadomasochism (SM) are the terms everyone knows, but a lot of people don't realize that the middle two letters stand for dominance and submission (DS).

The term started back in the 1990's and is used as a general term that includes a wide variety of activities and participants. Most BDSM groups welcome anyone who would identify as *kinky*.

The Scene – The scene refers to the world of kinky sex and BDSM.

A Scene – A scene would be the noun to describe any type of participation in BDSM activities by one or more people.

Playing – Playing would be the verb used to describe the action of a scene.

Head Space – Another name for being in top, bottom, dom or sub space.

Top Space/Bottom or Sub Space – Different types of mental states you might be in when involved in a scene.

Play Space/Dungeon – The area you create or go to play in. Your bedroom may be your *play space,* but you also might go to a public dungeon to play.

Power Exchange – Two or more people engaging in acts during which a partner will give another partner some amount of power, control and authority over them for a negotiated amount of time.

Dominant/Dom/Domme – The person who is in control in a consensual power exchange relationship.

Submissive/Sub – The person who gives up control in a consensual power exchange relationship.

Top – The person who is giving the pain/pleasure.

Bottom – The person receiving the pain/pleasure.

Master/Mistress – A more formal title taken by a dominant that is either used as a sign of respect by their partners or simply used as an honorific by the dominant (ex: Master Bob).

Slave– A more formal title taken by a submissive that is either used as a sign of commitment to a partner or simply used as a title by the submissive (ex: slave Joe).

Switch – Someone whose identity is fluid, switching back and forth between both dominant and submissive, top and bottom or master and slave.

Vanilla – Anyone who does not participate in kinky sex/BDSM.

Identify – How you perceive yourself in the scene and/or your sexuality (Ex: He identifies as a bisexual switch, She identifies as a queer master).

Power neutral – A term coined by Bo back in the early 90's to explain a relationship where kinky partners do not participate in a power exchange with each other, but may with people outside the relationship; they are often polyamorous and often both dominant or both submissive.

Polyamory – Literally meaning "many loves", polyamory is the act of having more than one intimate relationship at a time with all parties having full knowledge and consent of such. Also often referred to as "ethical non-monogamy", coined by the authors of the popular book *The Ethical Slut*.

Newbie/Novice – Someone who is new to the BDSM/Kink world.

Limits – The activities you negotiate with your partner(s) that either you will not do under any circumstances (hard limits) or might do, but only under certain circumstances that you've decided on (soft limits).

Edge Play – Any play that is considered to be on the edge of someone's limits. Also a generic term for play that many would consider more dangerous or taboo.

Negotiation – Communicating with your partner(s) on what you are interested in doing, like or not like, limits you may put on certain activies, what your safeword is, and anything else that goes into negotiating a scene or a relationship.

Aftercare – The time you spend processing, discussing, and reconnecting with your partner(s) after a scene.

Finding partners on Fetlife.com

One of the first things that I suggest everyone reading this book does is join a free website called FetLife.com. For lack of a better term, FetLife.com is the Facebook of BDSM.

When you join, you don't have to put up a picture or a bio, unless you want to. But if you are interested in meeting people, that would be a prerequisite.

The great thing about FetLife.com is that it is a real place where real people meet and share information. Anyone who is a real player in the scene is almost sure to be a member.

There are three main ways to use FetLife.com. First is to view people's profiles and make friends just like you would on any other social media service. Second is to use the events tab and find out where interesting events might be happening in your area, if you are interested in venturing out into the BDSM scene. Third and most important, there are literally thousands of groups on

FetLife.com that represent almost every fetish you can think of. These groups hold hundreds of thousands of posts that you can review and get important information from.

If you are a submissive newbie who is interested in daddy/little girl play, then you'll find a ton of groups for daddy/little girl play besides many newbie groups, not to mention submissive groups.

You can join that group and you can read interesting posts and gather knowledge, start your own posts to ask questions or comment on other people's threads and become part of the community.

Whatever you use it for, FetLife.com is a fantastic resource and way to meet real life or online friends that are interested in BDSM/Kinky Sex.

WARNING: no matter how good a place is, there are still jerks. I didn't say it was perfect, but it's the best of the online BDSM sites.

Local groups

Many areas, and certainly most large metropolitan areas, these days have some sort of group you can be part of if you are interested in meeting people in person.

Often there are what's called "munches", which are usually groups that get together at a restaurant in a vanilla establishment. Here you can meet and talk to other BDSM-friendly people in a low pressure, vanilla atmosphere. It's a great way to break the ice and just get to know some people you might want to become friends or even play with.

If you are lucky enough to live close to a larger area, you probably have a support group in your area that meets regularly. The first one of its kind is called TES, The Eulenspiegel Society, which I've been an emeritus board member of for many years. If you want to see what events and meetings a group might have, visit the TES website (*www.TES.org*) and take a look around.

You can find all these munches, groups, and meetings in the Fetlife.com events pages.

Conversion

For many of you, converting the willing is your path to BDSM happiness. You'd be surprised at how many people are interested these days. All you basically have to do is ask someone if they've read *Fifty Shades of Grey* and then see how they react; It's pretty easy from there.

Also, more people are noting their kinky interests on more vanilla dating sites. The site OKCupid.com is a good example of a place where it is common to find people mentioning their interest in BDSM. Again, simply mentioning your interest in *Fifty Shades of Grey* in your profile is a good way to attract the kind of person you are interested in.

Am I terrible because I have dirty thoughts?

A few times a year, I have the privilege to speak to Dr. Miro Gudelsky's human sexuality classes at CUNY.

I love speaking to college students. There is something intoxicating about the raw power of youth, the questions, the ceaseless curiosity, the fact that, for the most part, they still believe they can do anything. As cliché as it sounds, it's truly satisfying to be able to impart some of your wisdom and experiences to people so young and hungry for knowledge.

As an expert in alternative sexuality, I have spoken in front of many colleges and groups over the years and the one thing that stands out for me is "that moment". The moment that you realize something you said had a profound effect on someone else. That moment when you feel the collective energy of the room change. That moment when you see someone shift in their seat and swallow hard. It doesn't happen all the time, but when it does, it's special.

"That moment" happened for me one day when I answered the following question:

Am I terrible because I have dirty thoughts?

I spoke a little bit about fear and the fear of your own thoughts. The fear that has been instilled in you since you were young, telling you that your sexual thoughts are "bad" or "wrong", that you are "dirty" and "terrible" for thinking about those things.

I told the students that EVERYONE has thoughts like that. It's really just a matter of how honest you want to be. We've all had a dark moment or two with our sexuality. Some of us a lot more than others!

Whether it's fairly gentile, like when president Jimmy Carter admitted to "lust in his heart", all the way to fleeting thoughts of things so dark and wrong, illegal, and immoral that you are convinced that "you must be sick in the head and a horrible person" -- RELAX.

There is nothing wrong with you, because everyone has these thoughts.

Humans are complicated animals, and our sexuality is tied in with all kinds of strange things in our psyche. There is only a problem when we allow repressed and frightened members of society to feed us fear, guilt, and dogma and make us feel bad about ourselves for having nothing more than a sexual fantasy!

So what if you have a filthy thought? So what if you even might ACT on these thoughts?! Heaven forbid that you might consider going out and finding a partner that you can talk to or act out this thought/fantasy with in a consensual manner.

How dare you have pleasure!

And if your thought is nonconsensual, illegal, or would hurt others, then in the immortal words of Chris Rock, "JUST DON'T DO IT!"

Point is, just because you think it, doesn't mean you have to act on it. Nor does it mean you should worry that you might. We all have lots of crazy thoughts. How many times have you gotten so upset about someone or something that you banished them in your mind forever? That you wished them ill will or WORSE?

We all have those dark moments. However, we just don't ACT ON THEM, and, for the most part, we don't worry about them. We know it's normal to get angry and lose it for a minute. We know we would NEVER do the wrong things... we just think them.

Well, it's the same with sexuality. We tend to fetishize things for the very fact that they ARE wrong. That they are taboo, etc. If these thoughts are "safe, sane and consensual" then you can even go out and find someone that shares your predilections. If not, your fantasy can just stay up in the old mental rolodex to whip out when you are, "alone with yourself" or when you want to whisper something very naughty into someone's ear.

There are two kinds of people in this world.

1. People who admit to dirty thoughts and desires

2. Liars

COMMUNICATION

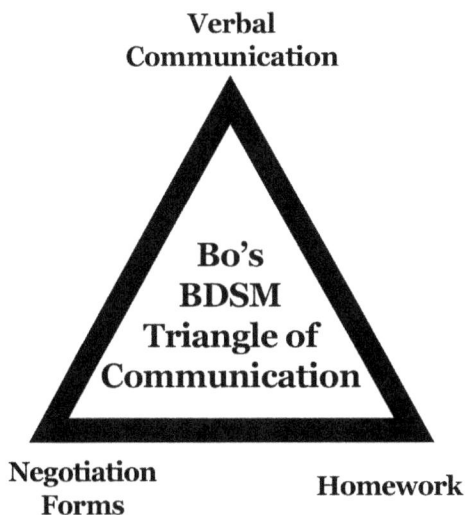

Verbal
Communication

Bo's
BDSM
Triangle of
Communication

Negotiation
Forms

Homework

Communication is one of my very favorite subjects. I've taught a class called *Communication, Communication, Communication* aka *Communication in the Scene* for many years. To help make it easy to remember the three main points of that class, I created *Bo's BDSM Triangle of Communication*.

Communication is the most important thing in any relationship, be it a vanilla (non-BDSM) relationship or a kinky one. The first point at the top of the triangle, is the most important, and we call this:

Clear and consistent verbal communication

You need to do your very best to learn to communicate with your partner verbally. For some this comes easily, and those of you who fit in this category are very lucky indeed.

For the majority of people, it's just not that simple. You may have spent your whole life being shy and having trouble asking for what you want in general, let alone in the bedroom. For many it is frightening to talk about fetishes or interest in kinky sex, worrying about being judged or misunderstood by partners and hearing the dreaded phrase:

"What are you, a freak?"

For many of you, this type of reaction is your worst fear realized. There is a very good reason many of you feel this way, we are socialized to be fearful and to be frightened of anything that does not fit society's conception of what is normal.

Luckily, I have created my super-duper, never fails, (well hardly ever) method for helping you and your partner communicate and I'm going to reveal it to you right now.

Wait until the two of you are in the mood to get sexy with each other. It doesn't really matter where, but a good place is when you are in bed together. Start touching your partner and begin to get them aroused. The goal is to get them excited and horny, not to have actual intercourse. Once you get your partner excited, congratulations... they will now be a lot more receptive to you talking about... well... just about anything! It's similar to when somebody has a drink, they loosen up a little bit. When you are horny, it is the same kind of thing and a good time to talk about something that is a little bit kinky or naughty.

You don't necessarily have to spring the whole thing on them right away, just get a conversation going. Ask them what kind of kinky things *they* might like. You might say something like:

> *"So, tell me, what is the kinkiest thing you ever fantasized about doing?"*

You want to let them know that *you really want to know*. Tell them:

> *"It makes me really excited to know what makes you excited."*

By doing this, you are opening up the lines of communication between the two of you. Reassure them. Give them as much positive feedback as possible, *that it's something you really want to know, it excites you to hear about it, and it will make you very happy for them to share this with you.* At this point, after you have asked them some of the things that they are interested in, you can tell them some of the things that you are interested in. By then they might be just as excited about this as you are!

Let them know if you are nervous, scared, embarrassed etc. Be honest. Let it all out. You might be amazed by the responses and reactions you get. Remind your partner that nothing that they fantasize about is wrong, it's just fantasy. Be prepared to hear some things you may have never expected. You need to create a judgment free zone. A safe place where you can say whatever you want.

The reality is most people want very much to please their partner(s), and if that is not where your relationship is at, you may want to reconsider if this is the right relationship for you. Sure, your relationship may be in a rut or you've stopped communicating well. There are always day-to-day stresses, fighting, children and bills, and all the other nonsense that makes relationships challenging. But, ultimately, partners want their partners to be happy, to be excited, to have good sex, and, of course, to come hard. It's usually just a matter of getting your partner in the right frame of mind to lose their inhibitions and not feel judgmental.

Unfortunately, sometimes this is easier said than done. I know you might find this shocking, but you may get some push back and resistance from your partner, *even while they are being lightly masturbated under the covers!* Hard to believe, I know.

Fear is a very powerful emotion, so realize that your partner may be so fearful of telling you their deep dark secrets that they may get angry during or especially after this type of thing. They may say, "I do not know what you are talking about. That is disgusting. That is terrible." Even tell you that you are "bad, sick or wrong for making me talk about this." Be ready for this possibility and be assured that *all is not lost!* A lifetime of being told these thoughts are dirty and wrong is a lot to overcome. Just keep reassuring and letting your partner know that it's just *fun in the bedroom.* However, you may need to try again at a different time or bring it up in another situation.

It is possible that some people may not feel open to things in a sexual situation, but feel better in a neutral situation where they can just talk about it. Know your partner, know the way they respond best, and work with that accordingly.

One of my favorite sayings, aka *Bo-isms,* is:

> *"I want to know everything about you so I can use it liberally against you."*

This is said with tongue in cheek, of course, but is actually very true. A dominant should strive for:

Relentless pursuit of information

Verbal communication is the easiest and quickest way to get information. Later on, we are going to explore some other ways for those who have trouble with communicating verbally to get information, but verbal communication is king.

This is not magic, this is simply having conversations, both vanilla and kinky. Sometimes they can be very direct, asking questions about what someone might be interested in sexually, and other times it's innocuous things that might be useful later on. Some common questions you can ask are:

- What are things that you've enjoyed in the past?

- What are things that you've fantasized about in the past but have maybe never done?

- What are the things you think about when you play with yourself?

This last questions is a very important one, and, again, sometimes very embarrassing for somebody to answer. You will often find that people have a core thing that they go to when they masturbate. Many people do not even realize that they do or, better put, they selectively ignore it. But a lot of people have a scenario, or particular fetish, that is a core thing they think about when they want to come or especially if they want to come quickly.

Use your imagination, as there are so many things you can ask. Get curious and turn it into a scene itself. It can be really hot to ask all these questions as if it's an interrogation or as light and fun humiliation play.

It is also not just sexual information that you are looking for, but almost any type of information, *because all information is good information.*

> *Some information can make you seem almost clairvoyant.*

It's impossible to remember everything, but the more information you can catalog in your brain and save for a rainy day, the better. After a while, you'll begin to realize what things are more interesting to remember than others. But just about anything could be something you might be able to use later on in a sexy scene with your partner.

For example, your partner might mention to you in a completely non-sexual conversation that *they were scared of the dark when they were a child and would always be afraid that something was going to grab them out of the darkness.* Many months later you might be having sex with your partner and ask them to put on a blindfold. Remembering what they told you, you won't be surprised at all to see them swallow hard and tentatively agree. You might then tell them that you are going strip them and tie them to the bed. Once you are finished, they will have forgotten that you know of their fear of the dark but you will remember and can create intensity by playing with these feelings. You might let your partner sit quietly for many minutes so that they start to worry that you might have left the room and then lightly touch them in various erotic areas every few minutes saying nothing and watching them react with a mixture of fear and arousal.

When we play with these fears we need to be extra careful to watch for our partners' mental states and make sure we are not pushing them too far. Later in this chapter we will discuss *safewords*, and you need to make sure your partner always has one, especially in this kind of situation.

Further gathering of knowledge leads us into the bottom of our triangle, where we have two different types of written information.

The first is called negotiation forms

They have been called many different things over the years, *negotiation forms, checklists, play forms, boundary lists, etc*, but they all basically do the same thing. A negotiation form at its core is just a way to find out the kinky things a partner *would, might* or absolutely *would not* be interested in exploring.

Usually, you are given a list of many different fetishes and types of play and are asked to rate them 0 through 5. Zero being an *absolutely not*, which is what is called a *hard limit* and means that *under no circumstances do you agree to do that activity*. All the way to number 5, that tells your partner that this is something you are very excited about doing or trying.

Often, the list will be quite lengthy and will give you several different types of terms for some of the same things. This is because different terms mean different things to different people.

On a good form there are usually some free form questions about health and safety, things you like the most or least, medication you might be on, old injuries etc. These are all important things to know when you engage in kinky play.

Negotiation forms can be very sterile. This is not like clear and consistent verbal communication where you are able to reply and ask for clarification or start a discussion. No matter what the form asks, you will only get answers based on the way your partner interpreted the information.

You might start by meeting someone new and using your verbal communication skills to talk about many different things. You might even have a little light play or foreplay, flirting, etc. and mutually realize that there is interest in taking things further. You might then email them a negotiation form, which will start the written communication process. The filled out form might lead to more verbal information about the form or even different types of written communication via email, etc.

Are you starting to see how this all gets put together and the magic of combining everything with our triangle?

And by the way, you can have someone fill out a negotiation form for you as a top or a bottom, dominant or submissive, no matter what you are interested in or how you identify, you can use these forms.

Remember, there are no rules in BDSM other than consent. These are all just great ideas for you to use to communicate with each other. You may find better or easier ways for you to do it with your partner.

Once you get your negotiation form back from your partner, there are a couple of things you can do with it.

You can read it, keep it to yourself, and never talk about it again. Sometimes, our partners are too embarrassed to write these things down that in order to get them to fill it out truthfully, you may have to tell them you'll never talk about it. And while that may seem funny or counterproductive, it is very true.

However, the best thing would be for you to read the form and find out as much information as you can and then, later, talk to your partner about it. One really fun way to do this would be, again, as foreplay with your partner in bed. It is a very sexy thing for you to discuss the different things that really excite you and here is a really good chance for you to clarify various things you've read in the form.

For a good example of this, let's look at one taboo subject-- *humiliation*. When some people think of the word humiliation, they think of it being something very degrading and powerful, tearing someone down to make them feel badly about themselves.

But what about a little sexy talk like:

"You are my little slut."

Your partner may like that very much but did not want to say so in the negotiation form, since they took it to mean degrading and tearing down, as opposed to playful.

So, again, this is a great time for you to gather more information and to quiz each other on things that you are unsure about. Essentially, when you look at these forms, you are looking hard at the 0's and 1's, and the 4's and 5's, as these give you the things your partner feels strongly about one way or another.

Certainly, sometimes just knowing somebody is interested in something to a moderate degree is important too. But, generally, wanting to know things that are absolutely great and absolutely bad are things that bring up the most important conversations.

To start off, you might look at the form and say:

"Gee, I see you put a 5 for tickling."

Which might be a bit mystifying to you as you never thought of tickling that way. So you might say:

"I do not even understand what you mean by tickling. You get excited by tickling?"

And your partner may tell you something you never knew: that for their whole life they've had a fantasy of being restrained and tickled.

To you, that may sound very silly, but to them it may be a life-long fetish that they want to explore. Remember, be careful and be kind here. Your partner may be telling you things that are deep dark secrets that they have never told anyone else in their entire life because no one has ever given them the opportunity to speak to them about it.

You have the opportunity to make this a wonderful experience or terrible experience for them. If you judge them or make them feel silly, they will probably shut down and never give you any more information or at least not for a very long time.

It's important to know that you do not have to like everything that they like or even be willing to participate. Going back to our example about tickling, you might feel that that is a very silly thing and you get nothing out of it. It does not excite you whatsoever, and you do not understand it. That is fine, but you still want to know.

However, in this example, where your partner told you that this was a #5 fetish and a lifelong fantasy, you will hopefully at least try to find some common ground here and maybe even find that it has become interesting to you. Maybe not because you ever fantasized about it before, but because you just found a way to make your partner extremely excited.

This is a very important concept. Playing around with games of dominance and submission are very much about knowledge and power. When you acquire knowledge about your partner, this can be used to heighten the sexual experience or the power dynamic.

So, your new excitement may be happening because you now know that you can make your partner react in a very extreme way with something that seems very innocuous and would not normally be something that you would have ever thought of.

We include a copy of our negotiation form here for you to review, but you can download it on our website in either a PDF or Word Doc format right now at:

www.50ShadesOfCurious.com/negotiation

==

50 Shades of Curious Negotiation Form

The more information you know about your partner, the safer and more exciting your playtime will be. Remember, communication is the key to all relationships, kinky and vanilla alike!

Below is a long list of KINKY/BDSM activities. Don't be overwhelmed by the list. You may have no idea what some of these things are, and that's OKAY! Some things might seem extreme or even shocking to you. Don't worry, you NEVER have to do anything you don't want to do. Sometimes we might only be interested in fantasizing about certain things and not actually doing them in real life. That's what negotiation is for, to share with your partner what you will, won't, and might do.

Take your time and answer as honestly and as best you can. Let the list give you new ideas, spur communication, and remember your answers will change over time and depending on what person you are filling this out for. Some words have similar meaning and are left ambiguous, to see what they mean to you. This form can be filled out by the top/dominant, bottom/submissive or switch!

Please put two to three answers next to each item:

The first answer should be, if you've ever tried that activity before

- Yes = I have participated in this activity before

- No = I have not participated in this activity before

The second answer should be your interest in engaging in that activity on a scale of
0 – 5, NO,?, +, ! or a combination.

- 0 = I have no interest/don't like this, but would do it to please you.

- 1 = Not very interesting/don't really enjoy this too much

- 2 = This is OK

- 3 = This is nice/fun/interesting

- 4 = I really enjoy/think I'll enjoy this activity

- 5 = I LOVE THIS/CAN'T WAIT TO TRY THIS

- NO = Hard limit. I will not participate in this activity at all, at this time

- ? = Unfamiliar with this activity

- + = I'm scared of this but would possibly like to explore it

- ! = I'm embarrassed to admit I like this

Examples:

Flogging: Yes/5 (Have done it before/LOVE IT!)

Biting: No/+ (Have never tried/scared of this but might like to try it)

Tickling: Yes/5+! (Have done this before/love it/scared of it/embarrassed I like it)

The third answer would be to write any explanations or more information after your answers. Remember, the more information you share, the safer/hotter/more fun things will be.

Examples:

Flogging: Yes/5 - I especially love to be flogged on my back!!!

Tickling: Yes/5+! - My feet are my most ticklish place but I didn't tell you that! <s>

==

Age Play:	Biting:
Anal Sex:	Body Modifications:
Arm/Leg Sleeves:	Bondage (heavy):
Begging/Pleading:	Bondage (light):
Being Blindfolded:	Boot Worship:
Being Gagged:	Breast Bondage:
Bestiality:	Breast Whipping:

Breath Play:	Face Slapping:
Brown Showers/Scat:	Fantasy Gang Rape:
Caning:	Fantasy Rape:
Chauffeuring:	Fire Play:
Choking:	Fisting:
Chosen Clothing for:	Flogging (back):
Chosen Food For:	Flogging (butt):
Clothespins:	Following Orders:
Cock Worship:	Foot Worship:
Collars (wearing):	Forced Dressing:
Corsets (wearing):	Forced Homosexuality:
Cutting:	Forced Masturbation:
Daddy Play:	Forced Nudity:
Double Penetration:	Forced Servitude:
Duct Tape:	Full Head Hoods:
Electricity:	Gags:
Enemas:	Genital Sex:
Examinations (physical):	Given Away:
Exhibitionism:	Golden Showers (piss play):

Hair Pulling:

Hairbrushes:

Hand Jobs:

Handcuffs (metal):

Harnessing:

Head (getting):

Head (giving):

High Heel Worship:

Homage With Tongue:

Hot Waxing:

Housework:

Human Pony:

Human Puppy:

Humiliation In Private:

Humiliation In Public:

Ice Cubes:

Including Others:

Infantilism:

Interrogations:

Intricate Rope Bondage:

Kicking:

Kidnapping:

Kneeling:

Knives:

Latex:

Leather Restraints:

Lecturing:

Licking:

Massage(getting):

Massage(giving):

Medical Scenes:

Mommy Play:

Mouth Bits:

Mummification (saran wrap:

Needle Play:

Nipple Torment:

Oral/Anal Play:

Orgasm Control:

Orgasm Denial:

Over-the-Knee Spanking:

Phone Sex:

Piercing (perm):

Piercing (temp):

Pony Play:

Punching (controlled):

Punching (beat down):

Pussy Whipping:

Pussy Worship:

Religious Scenes:

Riding Crops:

Rope:

Scratching:

Sensory Deprivation:

Serving as Ashtray:

Serving as Furniture:

Serving as Maid:

Serving Orally:

Serving Other:

Sex in Scene:

Sexual Deprivation:

Shaving:

Single Tail (light/sensual):

Single Tail (moderate/heavy)

Spanking:

Speculums (vaginal):

Spreader Bars:

Stocks:

Straight Jacket:

Strap-on Dildos:

Supplying Victims:

Suspension:

Swapping:

Swinging:

Taboo Themes:

Tattooing:

Teasing:

Tickling:

Triple Penetration:

Uniforms:

Verbal Humiliation:

Videoed Scenes:

Voyeurism:

Whipping (cat o' nine
etc.):

Wrestling:

==

Important Questions:

Physical Concerns - Do you have any medical conditions, chronic or otherwise, that the top should know about, such as epilepsy, weak shoulders, skin allergy, etc.? Are you on any prescription medications?

Mental Concerns - Do you have any phobias or mental conditions that the top should know about (fear of heights, claustrophobia, etc.)?

Limits - Are there any specific scene-related things you will not do?

Fetishes - Are there any specific scene-related things that you really like or dislike? Something that has not been mentioned above:

======================================

After you have discussed your negotiation form with your partner and read it yourself, you will have a lot more knowledge about what your partner likes, hates, wants, loves, etc.

This leads us to the third part of the triangle, which I call homework.

Homework is simply checking in with your partner after you have had playtime with them or enter into any activity that would be power, BDSM or kink related. What you decide should warrant a homework assignment is up to you and your partner, but anything other than your usual lovemaking may apply.

Once such an event occurs, you might say something like:

> *"I expect some homework on this. I want you to go home and write me an email telling me how you perceived what happened tonight."*

It is very important that you tell your partner that no matter what they say, you will not look at them badly or punish them in any way. If you do not do this, you will never get the information you want.

You will really need to have no ego here, if you can't do that then do not even bother. You will need to be ready to hear the cold, dark truth that your partner may not perceive the experience the same way you did.

It is a common occurrence for someone to come up with an idea for play time and then put a lot of time into thinking about it. Finally, the day comes to act out that scenario and they are naturally very excited about it. The play time unfolds and everything seems to have gone really well!

You request homework from your partner and when it comes you notice that there are thirteen paragraphs about some small little thing that you have not even planned to do and only a brief sentence about the actual thing you planned and worked so hard on.

Welcome to exploring the human sex drive, It can be very humbling, but if you can deal with the fact that maybe you are not always going to be

Master Great Grand Poohbah of All Space and Time

You can learn more than you'd have ever thought.

Let's say, again using the example from before, you were inadvertently tickling them during one part of your scene. When you get your homework back, if it has been done properly by someone who is not afraid that you are going to punish them or be disappointed in them, they will write something like:

> *"We did the scene, it was very fun. I have always had a tickling fetish. My partner tickled me for a few minutes and it was absolutely amazing. All I could think about for the next three days was how I wish they would have continued to tickle me until I was begging and pleading for them to stop."*

That is the kind of information that changes relationships. If you are willing to hear it, you will find information that can be extremely valuable. Remember, knowledge is power, and knowledge is safety.

Homework is the last part of the triangle of communication, and the three things together truly can be more than the sum of their parts. By combining all three and doing your very best to get as much information as possible, you will learn how, what, and why your partner desires what they do.

Negotiating

The negotiation form should not be confused with the act of negotiating. A negotiation form is one excellent way to negotiate, but there is more to negotiating then just a form.

Verbal communication is even more important than written communication in this situation. We want to talk to each other about what we want, not just write about it. Having a give-and-take conversation helps to build trust.

You want to do your best to tell your partner what it is you will and won't do, and to do that, we have to make sure we are on equal footing with each other. Meaning, don't negotiate with someone somewhere you feel too intimidated to talk freely. Perhaps when you walk into your partner's home, you immediately feel submissive and powerless to them. This is not a good place for you to negotiate. Go out to a coffee house, take a drive in the car, but make sure you are negotiating somewhere you feel equal and can accurately represent your concerns, fears, wants, and desires.

At its best, negotiating is a way for both of you to talk about what you each want. It's not just for the bottom, it's for the top too. This should be a chance to talk about your desires, fantasies, fetishes, and find common grounds.

Then, before you actually engage in a scene with someone, you'll want to negotiate that specific event. It's really impossible to negotiate everything that might happen in a scene, which is why we have safewords. Safewords help ensure that you can always stop a scene any time you need to and are discussed in the next chapter.

Here is an example of a negotiation you might have with someone you've never played with and don't know very well. You have spoken a bit and he's asked if you want to play. You've talked a bit about spanking and that he enjoys that and you think you will too.

So you might start out by limiting the play *only* to spanking. Saying that:

"You only agree to participate in a spanking scene."

Next you might want to negotiate the severity, so you'd say:

"I've haven't done this very often, so I'd prefer you don't go too hard, I'm still getting used to this."

Then thinking ahead you might add:

"My safeword is "RED, but if you put me over your knee it might be hard for you to hear my safeword, so if I grab your ankle consider that another safeword."

Your proposed partner might then ask:

"Are you interested in any touching or sensuality while we are playing?"

And you would then answer accordingly as to what you are interested in. Let's say you reply:

"Yes, that would be great."

You have now negotiated a nice simple scene, which:

- Will include spanking only
- Should not be too hard

- Can be sexy and include touching

And made sure that:

- Everyone knows both your safeword and safegrab

This is a well conducted negotiation where you both have input and you have both agreed to a scene. It's perfect for a simple scene. Of course, not everything will be so easy. You might be negotiating a much more complex scene and so a lot more discussion will be warranted.

NEVER make the mistake of just assuming that the person you are playing with knows what you want. Neither of you are mind readers, both parties are responsible to make sure the other knows what's important to each of you.

Also if you are playing with someone that you don't know well, it's a great idea to remove some of the role play element that could potentially require a safeword. You can role play to your heart's content when it comes to everything except consent.

You can be the teacher disciplining the student, you can be the naughty little girl who has displeased her uncle, you name it. But it's a great idea to remove the need to rely on safwords in the beginning and just say.

"Let's not role play with consent. If I say stop or ask you to change something, you need to do that please."

If you want to beg and say no, no, no, and not have your partner stop, there is plenty of time to do that in future scenes, after more trust is built. STILL MAKE SURE YOU HAVE A SAFWORD. Just in case your partner gets a little carried away you can still yell RED or SAFEWORD if there is *any* type of miscommunication.

As you play more with a partner or if you are playing with your boyfriend/girlfriend/spouse you will have more trust for your partner and feel more comfortable negotiating scenes with less restrictions. But regardless of your relationship with the person, you should negotiate until you feel completely comfortable with what's about to happen.

Often after playing with someone quite a bit, almost no negotiation needs to be done because you've negotiated all these things in the past and unless something has changed you already know what the rules are.

In that case you might only need to negotiate new activities or if you have changed your mind on something. It's common for you to come back to a partner and let them know that you are newly comfortable about a particular type of play and "since it went so well last time", you're comfortable with it being more intense OR maybe it was *too* intense last time and you need it to be different this time, etc.

Contracts

While contracts certainly are negotiating, they are usually more of a formal and fancy way to lay out the negotiated parameters of a more serious BDSM relationship.

Contracts are absolutely not needed. Quite obviously, real slavery was thankfully outlawed long ago so there is no legal element, and even though you might agree to certain terms in a contract and do your best to uphold them it's important to realize you can withdraw this consent at any time.

This said, having a contract between partners can be a deep and very important document that lays out your relationship and what is important to you.

What's in a contract varies greatly depending on what purpose it is serving. Contracts usually contain the hard limits of each participant, safewords, any promises or agreements that have been made and generally lay out the parameters of the relationship.

Sometimes contracts are just for a period of time, like a weekend or a month or some longer amount of time. Other contracts are more open ended like a marriage, and may have a clause that they are in force until one of the parties decide to terminate it.

Basically, contracts are a ceremonial way for you to lay out the parameters of what you'll both be responsible for in the relationship, both physically and emotionally.

CONSENT

BDSM cannot exist without consent. If there is no consent, then there is no BDSM. Rather, there is abuse. To be able to keep things consensual at all times, we have safewords.

Very often when we play with our partners, we find it fun to role play, and we say things like:

"No, stop, don't!"

Or something similar that may sound as if our playtime is not consensual.

When we role play, it is essential that our partners have a way to alert us that they need us to stop for real and that they are not just playing. Many people will tell you if you play with somebody who will not give you a safeword, you need to run away--

This is often VERY GOOD ADVICE!

However, it can also just be miscommunication.

I always say that if someone tells you that you don't need a safeword, simply ask them:

"Will you stop if I say stop?"

If they say anything other than "yes", RUN AWAY!

But if they do say yes, then they may not be interested in the power dynamic. They might be someone just interested in trying some things out together or they are not interested in role playing and are into a more sadistic or masochistic type of play. Either way, this means--

If you say stop, don't, or ouch, your partner will stop.

So in this case, the *safeword* is simply stop, don't or ouch, and a different word is unnecessary. It does not mean that the person is dangerous or there is anything wrong with that person. They are just not interested in playing with you in a role playing dynamic and will take you at your word, like they would at any other time.

However, we often like to play with at least a little role play. In the event that you do too, you must have a way to alert your partner that you need things to stop.

The moment that the scene becomes non-consensual is the moment the scene ends and abuse begins.

Obviously, we do not use the word stop or don't as a safeword when we *are* role playing, as those are the words that are the most fun to say.

The most common safeword is simply the word *Red*. Red is used the same way one would use a stop light:

- Green means go

- Yellow means slow down

- Red means stop

Some people like to use both yellow and red. Often they will say yellow when something is getting too intense or too scary, but they would rather not stop the scene completely.

Other people will use red for all things and just assume that you will check in with them as soon as they say red and decide if the scene will continue.

Other people will use funny words or words that would not come up in normal conversation. You might have someone who uses words such as elephant or chocolate teapot or any other odd word or phrase. Personally, I am not a big fan of this as, sometimes, when you are in the heat of a scene, it is very difficult for your partner to remember what the safeword is. This is not the time that a submissive or bottom wants their partner to have a problem remembering how to keep the scene consensual. The submissive or bottom want their partner to be able to quickly and easily stop things and check in.

The interesting thing about safewords is that your partner can often take a lot more of whatever it is that you are doing together when they have a safeword. Because, when these things are going on, they are able to say to themselves:

"Well, this is very intense but I know I can stop it if I need to."

Some use safewords as a way that they can play on the edge of their limits. They will play intensely with their partner until a safeword is said.

In the book *Fifty Shades of Grey*, there is a controversial scene at the end, between Christian and Anastasia. I quote Christian saying:

> *"For the record, you stood beside me knowing what I was going to do. You did not, at any time, ask me to stop. You did not use either safeword."*

This is a tricky situation and there is an excellent point to be made here that often there are a various chemicals going off in our brains and we are not always in our right minds when we are in a scene.

You may have heard terms like being in headspace or floating, which are sensations caused by the various chemicals flooding the brain as you get deeper and deeper into a scene.

The problem with Christian's comment is that it is still his responsibility to think for both people in the equation. He is not allowed to simply say:

> *"Well, you did not safeword so I am absolved of all responsibility."*

When someone is in deep headspace you could almost ask them to do anything and they would say yes. For example, if you said to your partner, "I am going to saw off your leg now," your partner might be in such deep headspace that they may actually look at you and say "Yes, do it."

Now, of course, you are NOT allowed to do it.

But, by Christian's remarks he feels that as long as no one is safewording that it is not his responsibility. So, you can see that this is a sticky wicket and sometimes can be a problem.

Everybody has to be part of the equation. And that brings us to another form of general scene communication, which is the BDSM motto:

Safe, sane, and consensual (SSC)

Consensual is always the most important. There must be consent between both parties. But, safe, sane, and consensual is saying that we need to play as safely as possible, be as safe as we can, and to be sane for all parties involved. In the above case, it is not sane nor safe to cut someone's leg off, so you cannot do that no matter how much consent there is. In this particular situation, this is not safe, sane, nor consensual.

This concept of sanity can also come into play when a partner becomes extremely stubborn, simply forgets their safeword or becomes confused and disoriented.

Looking back at the scene that Christian had with Anastasia, there is no way to know whether or not it would have been more appropriate for him to stop. We were not there. We cannot know from the book itself whether or not the consent and sanity were present.

He was trying to show her exactly what it was that he wanted, and she was prepared to receive it. However, it is very possible that Christian would have been better off going a bit easier on her.

Also, let us be very clear that Anastasia really does not seem to be very interested in pain. That is a huge thing here. She may be into following orders and pleasing her partner sexually in other ways, but she may really not be into corporal punishment, and that is absolutely fine. So, as a partner, Christian may need to pick up on that and simply say:

> *"I see that you are not interested in corporal play."*

The relationship may have to be adjusted or abandoned. We are not always compatible with everybody. And, although Anastasia may have fallen in love with Christian, she may truly not be interested in what Christian has to offer.

That said, she may also be very interested, but have a lifetime of socialization that is causing her to fight against it. My point to you is there is no clear-cut answer as to what should have happened in this situation.

Should Christian have stopped? Should Christian have continued? The questions can only be answered by the two partners and by considering what had been said in their complicated interactions.

Also, if you are going to participate in BDSM it's important to realize that:

BDSM is a contact sport.

BDSM subjects you to danger in a very similar way that playing tackle football or participating in the martial arts might expose you to.

It is very important for you to realize that sometimes things can go wrong.

Sometimes there can be both mental and physical injuries.

There is another acronym in the scene that is called RACK, which stands for "Risk Aware Consensual Kink". People who adhere to this motto believe that it's impossible to be completely safe, so you should at least be aware of the risk when you play.

Both have their merits, but RACK leaves out some important things, so I like combining them together and saying "Safe Sane Risk Aware Consensual Kink". It's not a sexy acronym, but we can all get aboard the "S.S. RACK" and sail away to safer BDSM.

Regardless of what you decide, it is crucial to think about what you are doing BEFORE something might go wrong.

Hopefully, with safewords and adherence to principles like SSC (Safe Sane Consensual) & RACK (Risk Aware Consensual Kink), we are able to mitigate most danger. But, you need to remember you can never eliminate it entirely.

Which brings us to three words that are near and dear to my heart: truth, integrity and honesty.

BDSM cannot work without truth, integrity, and honesty always being maintained. It is difficult enough to have a relationship in the vanilla world and keep that working, let alone in a relationship that includes kinky sex and role playing.

In our example above, Christian has decided to continue punishing Anastasia to a point that she is very upset. This is not necessarily a bad thing. Sometimes, this is exactly what the partner wants. Other times, it is exactly what the partner DOES NOT want.

It is very difficult to know what is right, but this has to be done by careful consideration and careful communication and observation of your partner. The point here is less is usually more. You are better off taking your time. There is always time to play again another day, and to go heavier, harder, and deeper.

In this case, perhaps, it may have been better for Christian to stop sooner when he saw the level of agitation in his partner, especially if his integrity was telling him that although he might be enjoying the reaction he was getting, it was not the one he had expected and his partner was probably not experiencing "good" pain.

Again, if it was the exact reaction he expected and his partner had completely agreed to it, and was well aware of her safeword, then that is a different story.

But, remember, your integrity is everything when it comes to playing around with *power*. The truth is, most respectable people who practice BDSM find that they rate their honor and integrity as the most important trait for them to possess.

How can you be in control of someone else if you cannot control yourself?

For example, a dominant would never take advantage of a situation when someone was drunk, because they should realize that the person is not in their correct state of mind.

This would correspond to the sanity portion of our safe, sane, and consensual discussion.

Being willing to be upfront about what you want in your relationship is another example. Telling someone in the beginning that you are married or that you are not interested in something serious or that you are polyamorous and never going to be interested in monogamy are all things that your integrity should be telling you that you must do.

Another one of my favorite sayings, aka *Bo-isms,* is:

> *"You have to be willing to lose to gain"*

In this example, you need to be able to say:

> *"Look, this is who I am, this is what I do, and if you are not interested then do not get into a relationship with me."*

People who have less integrity might think:

> *"Well, let me tell them this information later on when it is a better time or when they are bit more interested in me."*

If you do this then you are trying to trick and persuade someone and, in my eyes, that is not BDSM. That is abuse". You must carry yourself at the highest integrity at all times if you wish to participate in BDSM.

BDSM relationships are built on honesty and trust. It is important to remember that this trust is gained by integrity, consistency, and honesty, and is never taken, but earned.

You earn respect by showing you are trustworthy, by showing you have integrity, and by being consistent with that information over and over. That is the only way to build the trust of a partner. If you truly want to experience all this world has to offer, you must follow this advice.

Another example, as we discussed before, is taking advantage of people when they are not in their right frames of mind. When your partner is under the influence of the chemicals in their brain, drugs or alcohol is not the time to ask them to make decisions.

It's natural when you want something to wait for a good time to propose it to your partner. But there is a huge difference between a good and bad mood vs. an altered state.

Let's say your partner has said no to a certain activity every time you have ever asked them, and now, after a lovely night on the town, your extremely drunk partner is suddenly agreeing to the very thing she always says no to.

It's never easy, but the right thing to do is NOT act on this consent as it comes tainted. A person with integrity should say to themselves, "No matter what answer I get, I will make sure that the answer is the same tomorrow before I decide to take them seriously.

Often, we make rules in BDSM for various reasons. Perhaps you are playing with someone, but not dating them. You decide to keep sex separate and not have any in this relationship. You might have a dynamic where you just enjoy getting together and doing some spanking with your partner and that is all. You might tell your play partner that you are not going to have sex with them, that they should not expect it.

One day, after playing together for many months, you look at your partner a bit differently and realize you have gotten very excited and would like to have sex with them. The problem is that you've said you would not do that.

There is a huge difference between changing your mind and losing your integrity and changing a rule because you are becoming sexually excited and decided you want something badly.

Again, do not lock yourself in a corner. Rules are made to be changed, but not when you and your partner are in headspace, not when you are in the heat of the moment, and not when you are in the heat of pleasure.

You can make the same change of decision tomorrow and say:

"You know, we talked about not having sex together. I am going to change my mind, and I think that is now acceptable to have sex."

And as long as your partner is fine with that, then enjoy it.

RELATIONSHIPS

Romance

There are many types of relationships in BDSM. Some are more romantic, some less. Some people are just spicing up their sex life. Others are full-blown lifestylers, and there are many different types in between.

What one thing means to you may not mean the same to someone else. Remember the mantra, there are no rules in BDSM except for consent. Make sure you do what is right for you. What level of romance you want is up to you. For some people, BDSM is all about power and control and not about romance at all.

For many of you, you are reading this book to spice up your sex life with your existing partner. Hopefully, you already have romance in your life with that person and that romance will carry over into your play.

Be careful not to confuse romance with sex. You may have a lot of sex while you are roleplaying with your partner, but not have much romance; you'll decide whether or not you want the romance to spill over into your BDSM.

If you wish, you may decide to keep romance in your day-to-day vanilla life, but to have much less romance in your BDSM activities. You may decide that when you are participating in BDSM, or *playing*, one of you is the dominant and the other is the submissive, and it is purely about roleplaying. All you may be interested in is power and control, as well as giving and receiving the pain and pleasure.

There is no right answer here. You should do whatever you and your partner/partners wish to do. Also, you should feel free to change your mind from scene-to-scene and day-to-day. Sometimes, you may wish to play a more romantic style of BDSM, other time you may wish to be very cold and calculating and purposely remove the romance from the relationship. Feel free to do whatever works for you.

Let's take a look at the separation of romance and BDSM and why it might sometimes be desirable.

You may have partners that you are not in a romantic relationship with at all, but purely in a master-slave relationship. Perhaps they don't live together and only play together sometimes. If the slave sleeps over, in that type of situation, not sleeping together makes perfect sense. The relationship is more rooted in service and obedience than romance or sex.

Sleeping apart might also be something you do with your partner only when you are playing. You may actually be doing it as part of a *scene*. In your everyday life you can be very romantic and loving, sleeping together and spooning to your heart's content. But when the roleplaying/power dynamic starts, you might tell your partner something like:

> *"you are a slave and not allowed to sleep on the bed, you must sleep on the floor where you belong."*

This is an example of a type of role play you might do with your partner. This is not necessarily a common thing, but it is one example of the endless hot things you can play around with.

Often people separate sex from romance in BDSM. From one partner to another in a polyamorous relationship or even the way they might interact differently with their monogamous partner.

You may choose to have sex in your vanilla time together, but during your SM you may choose to not have sex or even be sensual. Again, it is all up to you. Sometimes, a person's interest in BDSM is not of a sexual nature, so their BDSM play will be strictly power and pain catharsis based. For others, it is very sexual.

In their head, a dominant might rationalize things by saying that they only *fuck* their slave, while *making love* is reserved for their partner. What is the difference? Sometimes very little in reality, but a lot mentally. Often people will reserve what they perceive as romantic sex for their partner, but still feel fine being *sexual* with their submissive(s) or play partners.

Some dominants don't have sex or play sexually with their submissives at all. For some people, BDSM is purely masochistic and sadistic. It is about giving and receiving pain in a cathartic way, and is not really sexual. It may be sexual later or something someone might think about when they are alone masturbating or with another partner. But often, it can be something that is non-sexual and purely a pain thing.

However, for the majority, BDSM is usually at least sensual if not sexual. While there may not be any active sex, there may be quite a bit of sensuality. It is common to see people playing out in the lifestyle scene and seeing no sexual contact whatsoever. All the sex happens later back home or not at all. When people are playing privately with a partner, it can often be more sexual as there is privacy and the opportunity for more sexual acts.

Also, getting back to the delineation, some dominants may set various different rules for their submissives or play partners. They may have different rules for different people. For example, they may know that they have a partner who is a hopeless romantic. But since that person is not their primary partner, they do not want to create a confusing environment. So they may choose to not have sex or even any sexual activity with this person. They may just enjoy some sensual play or none at all and stick to more cathartic pain play.

Some people just cannot do the polyamorous thing, and that is fine. So, if you are playing with someone who has other partners, you may need to keep that relationship non-sexual for you to feel good about it.

The daddy

The daddy/caretaker is a common reoccurring theme in BDSM. Both male and female can identify as daddy or mommy. The daddy dynamic in the scene can be anything from playful to extremely serious.

Again, there are no rules, just what floats your boat and is consensual. There are all types of daddies and all types of daddy play. You may wish to have a naughty dynamic, where you feel like your partner is your daddy. There are many taboos that this breaks, but many people find this very arousing.

There are also many people who adhere less strictly to the authentic daddy concept, but just play around with daddy ideas and iconography. For example, a male dominant calling his submissive little girl, is quite common.

A female submissive will often see a lot of similarity between her daddy/little girl dynamic with her partner and real paternal feelings she may have or, more importantly, wished she had about her real father, such as respect, obedience, love, affection, etc.

The daddy/little girl dynamic may or may not include a real father-daughter type role play. Many times, it is just a dynamic. Sometimes that includes what is called age play, where some people feel like they like to regress to a younger age. This is common because many people like to lose all responsibility and turn over power completely to someone else. This is something that is obviously done in the dominant/submissive dynamic as well, but can be done in a different, sometimes more intense way, with age play.

The punisher

The stereotypical view of BDSM play is that the dominant always uses pain as punishment, but you should know that not all relationships work that way in real life.

Punishment just won't work for some, since many people crave pain. Many use that pain for catharsis, and some need it like a drug. Others just enjoy it very much. For those relationships, pain is no longer punishment, but rather a reward. In these situations, the exact opposite is more effective. The removal of play and pain or removal of the dominant is how punishment is often given.

For example, a dominant may say:

> *"Because you have displeased me, you will leave and not be allowed to come back for a week. While you are away, I want you to think about what you have done and why you will never do it again."*

So, while some people can use pain for punishment, for other people it would just be giving the punished partner what they desire, and you can see how that would not work out.

Also, there are some submissives that would absolutely shrink at the thought of displeasing their dominant to the point of needing punishment. They may like pain for pleasure, but would be extremely upset if they had displeased their dominants. Many bottoms feel like they are good girls or good boys, and would feel terrible disappointing their dominant.

Just remember that there is a difference between bad punishment and good pain in BDSM. For some people, pain is a reward, for some people pain is a punishment, for some people pain is something they never want to ever receive because it would show that they had been bad. None of these are correct. They are all just different ways that you may express your dominance and submission.

Monogamous vs. polyamorous relationships

You will find both monogamous and polyamorous relationships in the BDSM world. They both can be very fulfilling, depending on what you are looking for.

For many of you, reading this book is all about expanding your existing monogamous relationship and you have absolutely no interest in any kind of polyamory, and this is wonderful. However, it may be something that you are interested in exploring. If it is

You need to know up front that, communication, honesty, and integrity are vital to the success of a polyamorous relationship.

There are many, many different flavors of polyamory. The word itself is a mash-up of the Greek word *poly*, meaning many, and the Latin word *amor*, meaning love. This leaves us with a very generic definition of *Many Loves,* which works just fine as the options under the polyamory umbrella are almost endless and are only limited by your imagination.

However you wish to live, your sex life should be up to you and your partner or partners. If it makes you happy and you all agree, then it's perfect for you.

The cliché of being in a relationship with other people where everyone is free to do whatever they want with whomever they want, whenever they want, does exist, but there are also many other types as well.

For some, polyamory may mean only for BDSM play, not for sex. For others, polyamory means three or more partners in an equal relationship that are all committed to each other and may or may not have other sexual partners.

Don't make the mistake of thinking that just because you identify as polyamorous—or poly—that you can't be in a committed relationship that includes fidelity. Not all polyamorous relationships are open to others sexually. They can just be three or more people who commit to each other or, for lack of a better phrase, consider themselves *married* to each other.

I have coined a phrase over the years called power neutral.

Power neutral describes one increasingly common polyamorous interaction in the BDSM scene, where a couple will decide they want to practice BDSM, but not with each other. In this kind of situation, both partners may be dominant or submissive or just not want a power exchange in their relationship, and they agree to get their BDSM play from others.

For example, if you are a dominant in a monogamous relationship, and your partner is dominant as well, it would be very difficult to ever enjoy a BDSM scene together, since you both like to be on the top. Some couples in this situation may just decide to be polyamorous, but only in certain agreed upon ways.

They may decide that they will scene with others so they can enjoy BDSM play, but not have romantic sex with others. They can create rules that work for them. Often, these rules may start out stricter and loosen over time as partners become more comfortable with the idea.

As I mentioned before, communication is so important here. It is crucial that you discuss your feelings, concerns, and interests with your partner(s), not once, but often, as feelings can change quickly.

You may begin as a monogamous couple who plays a little bit in the bedroom and progress to a couple that gets very, very interested in it and plays quite a bit. Then, one day, one of you tells the other:

"I might like to try playing with someone else."

This is a common situation and may or may not be okay with your partner(s). Clear and consistent communication is the only way to navigate these potentially treacherous waters.

The most important thing is to make sure your partner knows where they stand with you.

You want them to be assured that you love/care for them and that although there may be some difficult conversations ahead, it's to be expected. With all growth, there is some pain. And if you decide together that you may like to expand your sexual or BDSM activities to more than just the two of you, it's certainly going to take a lot of communicating.

Many people ask if swinging and polyamory are the same. They are usually not thought of as the same, but, in many ways, they are similar. They are both situations where people in a relationship add outsiders.

Those in a polyamorous relationship usually see themselves as people that are in a committed relationship, who engage in other committed relationships as well. Swingers tend to be people in committed relationship who get together for sexual activity with others.

Like most things in the BDSM world, semantics place a big part here. There are many polyamorous people who act like swingers, and swingers who act like polyamorous people, and everything in between. It is often how you may perceive yourself. Some people perceive themselves more as a swinger, some more as polyamorous, and others really do not see much distinction at all.

Just like BDSM, you should use the terms that work for you. Some people feel that swinger has a negative connotation to it, and that swingers are more interested in hedonistic, meaningless sex. Whether or not this is accurate to some degree, it does not mean that there is anything wrong with it. The reality is, it is all about doing what is right for you. What you call it is purely up to you and a necessary evil so you can explain to others what you are into.

Collaring and ownership

Obviously, there is no true *ownership*. Slavery was, thankfully, abolished many years ago.

In the scene, when people talk about ownership, slavery and collaring, they are talking about a submissive state of mind, a state of mind where you will let go and let someone else do the driving. You have committed yourself to that person in whatever form you choose. For some, that may be just once in a while in the bedroom when you decide. For others, it can be 24/7, day after day for the rest of your life.

Collaring and ownership mean different things to different people, but in most cases when someone says they are owned or collared they are letting you know that they consider themselves in a more serious, committed relationship.

Falling in love with your slave and 24/7 relationships

Of all the things in the world of BDSM, perhaps nothing is more precarious than the thought of living in a 24/7 relationship with someone. For many of you, you will be working backwards. You already may be in love with the person that you are interested in playing with and will be implementing BDSM into an existing relationship. For others, you may be in a BDSM relationship and falling in love with your partner. Both situations basically meet at the same place, so the question is how do you have a power relationship with someone and keep that dynamic alive when you love and care for them in a romantic way as well?

A great example of this can be found in *Fifty Shades of Grey*. As the book goes on, Christian may not realize it, but he is certainly looking at Anastasia differently than anyone he has looked at before. He is looking at her as a possible girlfriend. This is the beginning of some big decisions for him and the two of them as a couple.

It is almost impossible to have a true 24/7 fulltime, no time outs, BDSM relationship. Everyone needs some down time. No one can be *on,* always and forever. You could certainly play that way for a period of time. You can play 24/7 for a day, a weekend, maybe even a week or more. But there are definite things that need to be considered for anything more than that.

When will they have down time, and be power neutral? Will they constantly be in a power dynamic and will the bottom have to request *time out* when they need to speak as equals? Will they pick certain days of the week or certain places to be power neutral? Maybe they will just be kinky in the bedroom and power neutral in public? Perhaps kinky only at times they decide? Only on every other Sunday? Maybe they'll switch and take turns submitting every other week? The possibilities are endless.

> *"I thought you didn't let anyone sleep in your bed?"*

In the book, Christian has never let anyone sleep in his bed before and starts to allow Anastasia to do so. It's at this point that the internal struggle of 24/7 begins. Anastasia is questioning Christian's power. She honestly would like to know why he has changed his mind and has allowed her to sleep with him.

This is a very important thing if you are going to become more than just casual play partners. Consistency is very important. When someone is playing the role of the dominant, they need to be consistent.

Although the book is fiction and not about real people, It seems to me the author is telling us that Christian is becoming more comfortable with the idea of someone sleeping in his bed. Truthfully, Christian's sleep rules are probably more pathology than predilection. So, in this case, it is really just Christian healing a bit and feeling safe with someone sleeping in his bed.

But, if Christian had purely been doing this because he had made a decision in the past, then this would be an interesting situation worthy of further discussion, as it would appear that Christian is changing his mind on a whim. While changing your mind on a whim is perfectly acceptable for a dominant, it may also show a lack of integrity.

As a dominant, it's important to not to be so tight in your rules that you do not have any fun. You reserve the right to change your mind. This should not be confused with having integrity. Integrity is one of the most important things in the world of BDSM. We are playing around with some very intense mental and physical things here, so we truly need to have an amazing amount of it. But, there is a big difference between having no integrity and changing your mind.

My own rule for this kind of situation is simple: never change a rule or do something that might compromise your integrity in the heat of the moment. For example, perhaps you decided that no one is allowed to sleep in your bed because you don't want to confuse romance with dominance. Maybe you know yourself well and realize that after a night of sleeping together, you might begin to have a hard time separating the two and for whatever reason that is important to you. Then, one night, after a very sensual scene, you look at your partner in a whole new way and decide to have them sleep in your bed, knowing that it will lead to a sexy night of lovemaking.

Changing your mind at this moment is probably NOT a good idea because you are obviously making the decision in a compromised mental state. Your whole reason for putting in the rule was to keep you from doing something like this in the heat of the moment.

However, if you are home one night and call your play partner up and say, "I have thought about our no sleeping together rule that I imposed and I wanted you to know that I'm considering changing my mind on that as I think our relationship might be going to a different level. What are your thoughts?" that is a whole different story!

The point is, as long as you are changing your mind with integrity, growing and changing are two of the greatest parts about being kinky. You want to grow, so give yourself the room and permission to do so, just make sure you're making the decision in the right state of mind and for the right reason.

It is really not easy or common to have a relationship with a partner as both a boyfriend/spouse and a dom/master, and have no down time. Sometimes you want to act silly and playful. This is completely normal and fine. It is almost impossible to be the strict disciplinarian dominant every minute of every day of every year, nor is it even appealing.

Many dominants and, I would even dare to say, most dominants, as they become more comfortable in their dominance, have less and less trouble expressing their humanity and feel comfortable having time when they are power neutral with their partners. It is usually a beginning dominant that feels they must have an extreme amount of control to the point of even sometimes having no fun themselves.

If there is no down time, one can understandably jump to the conclusion that a relationship is abusive. Again, playing this strictly for a period of time is a tremendous amount of fun, but the thought of endlessly for the rest of your life, being controlled 100 percent at all moments is not only unrealistic, it is exhausting for the dominant.

When you hear someone saying that they are in the 24/7 total power exchange, what they usually mean is that they are living together or are together most often, and there is always a deference to the dominant, there is always a dynamic of dominance. But thinking that every minute of the day there is this serious overbearing dominance is very rare and pretty impossible to keep over a long period of time. If you hear that someone is in this type of relationship, it is very possible that they are in an abusive relationship, not a consensual power exchange. There are certain unique situations where people are in such relationships, but again, they are very rare.

However, it can be something done for short period of time as a scene. Actually, a weekend is perfect. Playing in a total power exchange for an entire weekend can be very demanding and exhausting, but a tremendous amount of fun.

Once the weekend is over, the power exchange is over and you can go back to your normal dynamic. Again, remember, the level of a power dynamic is completely up to you.

For example, you might be in an, up till now, vanilla/power neutral/equal relationship with your partner and decide that one of you is going to be the dominant and the other partner is going to be the slave for the entire weekend and do everything they are told unless they say their safeword.

That could be an extremely exciting idea. It could also only be for a day or just a few hours. But the idea of a couple who are in love with each other, trying out this type of power exchange for a certain period of time is completely different than an endless power exchange, where there is no hope of equality in the future.

Partners can create entire scenarios and games surrounding this kind of situation. Again, it does not have to be a complete power exchange. You may decide that you will be *daddy and his little girl* for the entire weekend. You may decide that you are going to be a *prisoner kept chained to the bed for one day.* You may decide that you are a *naughty schoolgirl with her principal at detention for the next three hours.* The scenarios are endless, and whether they last for a few minutes, a few days or even as long as a week or two, they are all just fantasies that are being played out for your mutual enjoyment.

Getting back to Christian and Anastasia, Christian is trying to make sense of everything and says:

> *"[T]he only time you do assume the correct demeanor for a sub is in the playroom. It seems that is the only place where you will let me exercise proper control over you and the only place you do as you are told."*

And perhaps, that *is* the only place Anastasia should assume the correct demeanor. What is developing between Christian and Anastasia in the book is a relationship in which Anastasia wants to be a submissive to her master, but only within the context of BDSM and the bedroom. For an existing couple trying to spice up there love life

This is likely the most realistic way for you to add BDSM to your world.

Your partner is your equal and that should not change in your day-to-day relationship. However, you do wish to relinquish that equality in certain situations and for certain time periods in order to enjoy the many benefits of a power relationship.

Enjoying casual BDSM with a partner is NOT about one person taking over complete control of the others life and bossing them around. You don't get to be automatically always right or get everything your way all the time. You certainly don't now have a license to hit your partner when you get angry or things don't go your way! You may role play like this all you like, if that's what you both want, but only in the times and places you designate together as *play time.*

Christian comes from a damaged background, and he thinks that he wants total control 24/7 in his partner's life. As he is learning from Anastasia, what he really may want is someone strong enough to stand up to him and be his equal in his day-to-day life, however, he may also want someone that enjoys relinquishing power in the bedroom and in the playroom.

Relationship advice

Remember, whatever relationship you are in, the best advice I can give you is:

You have to be willing to lose to gain

People tend to want to play things SAFE. To try to keep control. They'd often rather lose a little integrity vs. lose their relationship.

In a relationship you must be willing to lose that relationship in order to make it better and better. If your primary feeling is fear, you are in trouble. Not only are you being a phony, but your partner will not respect you.

This manifests itself in many ways, but most commonly by not revealing/discussing anything that you think might upset your partner and make them like you less.

Like the fact that you are kinky or want to be polyamorous or want to find a dominant partner and will really never be happy sexually otherwise.

This is great for the short term, but eventually everything comes out and not only the thing you were hiding, but your attempt to hide it itself. Even when it does not come out, it leaves you feeling bad about it and the energy you put out is "ugly".

You feel like a fraud, and you are.

People are attracted to confidence, honesty, and integrity. Sure it's easier to agree with your partner about everything. To make them think the two of you are perfect together. But really, you are just setting yourself up for a big fall.

Just be YOU and let the chips fall where they may. You do not HAVE to be perfect or exactly matched for someone to love you.

As a case in point, my wife and I are so NOT alike that it's comical. We don't like the same music, movies, food, friends, etc. BUT after 15+ years we are happier than ever.

The secret is our core beliefs are very aligned, most important is that we like time to ourselves. We don't LIKE to be together all the time. It suffocates us both. So for us... our mismatch is the perfect match!

To be clear, this does NOT mean you should meet someone and give them a list of everything you like and don't like. Also, many things change over time and you may not even KNOW how you are going to feel about something in the future.

No, this just means stop being SCARED TO BE YOURSELF. Have the integrity to speak your mind when you feel strongly about something and be just as willing to listen to others.

Being yourself, yet being open to growth and change, is the best way to enjoy life in my opinion. Life is too short to go around and worry if everyone agrees with you.

If you have a big topic to bring to your partner, this is often best left for a neutral time and not in the heat of the moment. This doesn't mean you have a license to put things off indefinitely. To be fair to you and your partner, you need to discuss this kind of thing BEFORE major decisions are made, not after, and shouldn't put it off just because you are scared things won't go your way.

Do you see a recurring theme?

FEAR = BAD

Getting rid of fear is easier said than done, but I urge you to boldly seek the truth and live an authentic life!

YOUR IDENTITY

One of the greatest things about the BDSM world is that, at its best, it is so welcoming and opening to every type of person of every persuasion, male, female, transgendered, queer, top, bottom, submissive, slave, dominant, daddy, master, owner, gay, straight, bisexual, switch, you name the persuasion and it is welcomed in this world. There is no right or wrong way to identify. You should feel comfortable identifying however you wish and also feel comfortable changing your identity as you see fit.

Indeed, this is one of the goals of the oldest BDSM education and support group in the United States, TES. I am proud to be an emeritus board member of the organization and have facilitated its novice group for over 10 years. One of my favorite things about the organization is its creed, which I include here in full; I hope you find it as inspiring as I do:

TES is a not-for-profit corporation which began as an informal association in the winter of 1971. We support sexual liberation as a basic requirement of a truly free society. Our special concern is freedom for sexual minorities and particularly the rights of those whose sexuality embraces D/s or dominant/submissive fantasies and urges.

These rights have largely been denied through negative public attitudes, internalized to a great extent by those possessing such inclination themselves. We assert the following rights for all:

- The right to pursue joy and happiness in one's own evolving nature, as long as this doesn't infringe upon the similar rights of others.

- The right to define oneself, and not be defined by persons whose experiences have not provided them with the understanding to appreciate one's mystique nor by those whose repressed urges may panic them into rigid hostility toward it.

- The right freely to communicate and socialize with others of similar sexual orientation, and to explore together the deeper, positive meaning of our experiences.

- The right to challenge established value systems which oppress by condemning and repressing sexual drives or practices of erotic minorities.

- The right to publicize activities and views - freely, without fear of occupational or professional repercussion-thereby raising the consciousness of both the public and ourselves regarding sexual or gender minorities and sexual freedom.

To realize these rights, we seek to foster consciousness raising and understanding among our members and the public at large through public forums and workshops on D/s, advertising, dissemination of Society publications and literature, by providing speakers for all forms of media, colleges and other audiences, and by giving support to other sexual liberation movements.

Most of all, we extend to our brothers and sisters who may be, as we once were, isolated, repressed and frustrated, the word that they are not alone, that a Society exists for them - straight, gay, lesbian, bisexual, transgender, and queer, all working together, with understanding and warmth, against misunderstandings and stereotypes, for freedom and fulfillment.

These words were written in 1971 by Pat Bond, the founder of TES, and they are as true today as they were then. I especially feel strongly about the right to define oneself not be defined by someone else who has not had the same experiences that you have had in your life. I truly think it is essential for your maturation that you consistently question and look at who you are. You should feel comfortable trying different things and changing your definition of yourself as often as you feel that you want to, so that you can grow as a person.

If you begin in a committed relationship, you may decide that you want to explore polyamory or if you are a top, you may decide you want to try bottoming or even switching back and forth. Maybe you want to wear diapers or dress androgynously, or perhaps you identify as heterosexual, but yet you may become attracted to someone of the same sex, etc.

Please do not feel intimidated to try different things. Do not feel that somehow it attacks some stereotypical role you are supposed to portray in society or in the BDSM world. The whole point of alternative sexuality is to shed all those preconceived notions and stigmas and to just enjoy yourself and go on a journey and see what happens.

I hope that you will explore. I hope that instead of possibly feeling stuck or influenced by your former vanilla life, where this kind of experimentation might be frowned upon, you will look at adding BDSM and kinky sex to your lifestyle as a way to grow as a person and be open to just about anything. You may very well find out that you are just as you thought you were, a heterosexual top or a submissive bisexual, or a gay switch or however you've identified over the years.

Also, be open to the reality that you may feel a different way with different people. You may be submissive your whole life and then one day you meet the one person who makes you feel extremely dominant. This is very common, and you should not be denying yourself the pleasure of a new exciting interaction with another person because of a stigma that you hold. Never say never, you may just surprise yourself one day.

When you are new it's very important to keep yourself open to new things or you are going to miss a lot of great stuff. Do not take the first person, including me, who tells you, "This is how it is," and just decide *that's it*. Bo says it is like this, so it is like this. I hope by now I've properly drilled into your head the mantra "there are no rules other than consent". Because, the whole point of the scene is to have experiences. That is the beauty of BDSM. This is a way to grow as a person. Find yourself, grow some more. Rinse and repeat.

But I'm so dominant in my life, don't I have to be dominant in the bedroom?

One has nothing to do with the other. If you have a type A personality and run everything in your vanilla life, that does not mean that you are going to be dominant in your sex life.

Your bedroom life can be very, very different from your day-to-day vanilla life. You will often find in this word that the people who are most dominant in their day-to-day lives are actually often the opposite in their sex lives. It is the typical yin and yang thought process. No one can be all one way or the other, there is usually a little bit of each.

There are certainly many people who are also dominant all the time or submissive all the time. This can just be the way you are wired, BUT, it also could mean that you need to take a hard look at yourself in the mirror to see if there are issues with your own self-worth.

For example, are you just scared to admit that you are insecure and have a deep need to be seen as a master or dominant? Do you have a terrible self-image and just feel like you don't deserve power and should always be submissive, in life and in the bedroom?

If you see some of this, don't worry, it doesn't mean that you don't get to identify the way you want. It does mean that you should work hard to work through these feelings and grow as a person.

If you realize you are an insecure dominant, then work hard to become a secure one. Many dominants start that way, the good ones grow into confident, powerful play partners.

You see, BDSM, is really just playing "pretend" in a very adult way. So, if sexually you enjoy being submissive, but realize it might not be for exactly the best reason, that's ok. This stuff about fetishes and such is complicated stuff. It's not even necessarily important to know why. But it can be liberating to examine your motives as sometimes that can help you grow tremendously as a person.

This all said, maybe you just want to have a good time spanking your partner before you have sex and this is all overkill for you. Remember the mantra: There are no rules in BDSM except for consent.

It cannot be stressed enough. There is no right way to do things. Take this information and do whatever you wish with it. It may apply and may not. But it's good to understand it, either way.

So are you implying that a dominant should consider trying the submissive side?

Definitely maybe! It depends on you.

For example, many years ago in the BDSM world, in what we now call the *old guard,* you would almost always have to start as a submissive and earn your leathers to become a master. You could not just decide you felt like a top, you had to start from the proverbial bottom.

Our BDSM history is rich and filled with tradition and wonderful things to keep alive, review, and learn from. However, there are also many different things that come out of the BDSM past that may no longer serve us, such as this outdated "bottom up" policy.

There is nothing wrong, and a lot very right, with trying the other side of the fence. But it is also important to know that doing so is not necessary. You are who you are. If in the beginning you feel submissive to people, this is a wonderful way for you to learn and acquire a tremendous amount of empathy for what other submissives go through.

Being a submissive when you start out can teach you valuable lessons. However, if you really are not submissive and have no interest in being submissive, then being submissive before you are dominant because it is required of you is foolish.

First of all, one cannot tell how something feels on someone else, only how it feels on themselves. Your empathy is limited. For example, you have a high pain tolerance while many others have a low pain tolerance or you have a certain fetish for something and others do not.

If starting out as a bottom or submissive feels right to you and that is the path you wish to take, then it's an excellent way to go, but it is certainly not necessary.

Also, if you are in a monogamous relationship with your significant other, the same holds true. If you just do not feel submissive then do not be submissive. However, being switchy with your partner, switching back and forth between roles, can be a wonderful way for two or more partners to coexist.

In a monogamous kinky relationship where there are only two partners, you are able to try more things than if one of you were just dominant and one of you were just submissive.

The most important thing is for you not to feel like you are bad or wrong because you do not want to be dominant, submissive or switch. You should be however you want to be.

Yet, be open to the fact that somewhere down the line you may decide to change. You may wish to be dominant for many years, and then eventually say, "I really want to try being submissive". Or you may say, "I am always dominant, but I really like how it feels when I am spanked. So, I would to like to bottom to somebody. I do not want to lose control or lose power, but I do want to feel pain."

There are so many different ways that you can go about it. There are so many different ways you can identify.

And the various words we use to try to explain how we feel are just language, used to try to help us communicate to others what we like or what we do.

It is important to see it that way, that it is just language, it is not who you are. You are whoever you are. These are just words to try to help us describe who you are. If you are a dominant, yet want to be spanked all the time, who is anyone to tell you that that is wrong. If you want to identify as submissive, but boss around your master, and that is good for them as well, then that is wonderful.

But why am I like this?

What does it matter? As long as it is consensual and you and your partners are getting what you want out of it, then enjoy it.

Many people argue that we are into this because of abuse in our past. Unfortunately, sexual abuse is a dirty little secret in this world that the powers that be frequently try to sweep under the rug.

Studies have said that anywhere from 20-60 percent of the population have been sexually abused. So while it would be nice to try to make a correlation, since anywhere from one-fourth to one-half of the population is being molested, it's a fruitless endeavor.

Instead, all that's happening is a huge amount of people with various fantasies are feeling very guilty about sexualizing some abuse from their past.

I say do not be abused twice. Whatever happened in your past, if you were abused, it was a heinous act, it was wrong, it was not your fault, and it was abuse. Now as an adult, if you sexualized it, you have three choices.

First, if you think that these feelings are interrupting your life, if you feel that these fetishes are keeping you from a productive life, then you need to seek some professional help. Just about all of us could do well to speak to a therapist or a psychiatrist to work out feelings, it helps you grow and become a better person.

Second, you can feel shameful and bad about yourself that you would sexualize something bad that happened to you, but you would just be victimizing yourself all over again.

Or third, you can simply not allow yourself to be abused again. If something turns you on, who cares why, unless it is interrupting a normal life. Remember, now you are doing this as an adult, and you are choosing to do it for play.

There is a whole type of therapy, called play therapy, that reenacts trauma to gain control over it. I am not going to say that you want to look at it as a way to heal yourself and subject yourself to it if does not excite you. But if it does, that can be a wonderful benefit.

The main thing is do not be shamed into pushing the thoughts out of your head. Simply enjoy them, especially if they are just something you masturbate to and not something you want to act out with your partner.

There are some things that are too powerful, intense, illegal, and immoral for you to do. So, just do them in your head, either while you are alone masturbating or when talking sexy with your partner, this is all good stuff.

The reality is, we have many different types of thoughts in our head, and there is a huge difference between doing those things and thinking about them.

So please, do not let yourself get abused twice. If you sexualized something from your past that was a dark bad thing, do not allow yourself to feel guilty about deriving pleasure from it now or, conversely, feel pressured to participate if you don't. Your choice.

How far should I go?

That's something you'll have to answer for yourself, but allow me to give you some advice. In *Fifty Shades of Grey*, Christian wants what he calls a true *24/7, full-time power exchange*. This is a master-slave type relationship where the submissive is controlled in all things - business, personal, and otherwise, are all taken care of by the dominant.

The truth is, this is mostly a fantasy and usually abusive if it's attempted in real life. Yes, if you are a billionaire like Christian Grey and can pay for everything AND put money away into an account for your partner's future as well, then maybe... but still only maybe.

The mental toll of a 24/7 is huge, especially if it's in a super controlled, master-slave type relationship.

It's also rarely fun for the Dominant either. It takes a lot of energy just to take care of yourself, let alone doing all the thinking for an entire other person, every day of every week, all year long.

What is much, MUCH more common is one of two other types of relationships.

The first is where the power happens strictly in the bedroom, during playtime, in the dungeon, etc. You are always equal and power neutral when you interact anywhere else. There is no power dynamic whatsoever outside play time.

Sometimes you might PRETEND to be in a 24/7 lifestyle for a scene, or a day or a weekend etc., but that would just be an extended play time.

However, if you would like to be in a more intense relationship with your partner, but don't want to get into a possibly abusive 24/7, all-consuming type thing, then the second type would be what I call *realistic 24/7*.

What this means is probably best explained by thinking about what it would be like living as a 17 year old in an idealized traditional family unit type household. If you lived in this perfect home, you'd be free to go to school or work and be encouraged to be the best you can be. Your parents would nurture and love you and want you to be happy. You'd have friends and go out with them when the family wasn't doing anything. If something bad happened, your parents would be there to counsel you and protect you. You'd have rules set for you and if these rules were hard for you to follow or too restrictive, you'd have the ability to go to your parents and ask to talk to them about it. They'd have final say, but you could go to them with your problems or concerns.

However, when dad or mom called, you would have to jump and do what they said. If they wanted the lawn mowed, it would get mowed, not later... but NOW. You would have respect for your parents and defer to them in just about any matter. You would never disrespect them to others or embarrass them in any way. You might certainly playfully tease them, but you'd know where the line was and wouldn't cross it.

Many people are attracted to this kind of arrangement. There are even people who take my example literally and have a "daddy/girl or boy" type dynamic with their partners. Either way, what you'd be having is a negotiable, safe, sane, consensual relationship with the loving illusion of being a real slave. There is something very compelling for many to be able to turn their brain off in certain areas and simply say, "my partner is taking care of it." If this is what you and your partner mutually want then it can be a very attractive model indeed.

If you are determined to go the full 24/7 route, I beg you to make some friends in the community and talk to other slaves so you can understand the reality of the situation BEFORE you commit to it. This is not something to get involved in lightly.

So what does it mean to be someone's sub/submissive?

Agreeing to be someone's sub can mean many different things to many different people. Remember, you need to define what that is to you. If your partner says, "do you want to be my submissive?" you need to turn around to your partner and say, "What does that mean to you?" One person's submissive is another person's slave, and one person's slave is another person's submissive. Roles can be widely different things to different people, and you need to make sure that you communicate a tremendous amount with your partner and confirm what these things are under a neutral power dynamic. Never negotiate things in a dominant-submissive or a master-slave headspace.

So, do a slave and submissive mean the same thing?

For some people, the answer is yes as they don't make any distinction between the two. However, I'd say that most people would consider a slave to be someone that is in a more serious, formal or committed power relationship. They may have signed a contract or been given a ceremonial collar to wear, or consider themselves to be the *property* of their master or mistress.

Conversely, *submissive* could refer to anybody who likes to play a submissive role. It could also refer to someone in a less intense relationship with a dominant or master. So most slaves would consider themselves submissive, but not all submissives would consider themselves slaves.

Just to be a bit more confusing, some people refer to themselves as Master Joe or Mistress Jane, but they are not necessarily YOUR Master or Mistress... confusing, isn't it? Again, no one is right or wrong. It's just how they decide to make it work for them!

Welcome to semantics and the world of BDSM.

We seem to have a never ending list of terms and words we use to describe ourselves and what we do.

Submissive, slave, switch, play partner, under consideration, collared, top, bottom, dom, domme, master, mistress, daddy, are all examples of terms that are used to identify people in the world of BDSM.

Although there are many different offshoots, the most common identities would be either switch, submissive/bottom or dominant/top. Many people believe that dominant and top or submissive and bottom mean the same thing.

Sometimes it does, and sometimes it doesn't. It completely depends on who you are talking with and how they interpret those words. I will say that for the majority of people who are active in a BDSM community, these words are NOT the same.

A relationship that includes role play usually uses the term dominant or submissive. Meaning that you are dominant and dominating your submissive partner. The reason we say that is *dominant* denotes power: you are dominant *over* your partner or submissive *to* your partner.

However, the designations of top or bottom often refer to the role someone plays in their relationship, not to the actual power or role play.

You may be a top, meaning you enjoy being the person in charge of the scene. Maybe you enjoy being a sadist and inflecting some sort of pain, discomfort, or even just giving intense pleasure. If you are a bottom, you are simply the one who likes to receive the pain, pleasure or the play.

These terms are often combined so that between the four topics, you can easily designate between the different ways that people identify.

You may have someone who feels that they are dominant, but they decided today that they are going to bottom to a friend. That may sound very strange, but is very common.

Remember that there are no rules in BDSM. You may have someone who is dominant in everything they do including in their sex life, but they also happen to enjoy pain.

They never feel that they give up their power. As a matter of fact, very often, you may find somebody who is a dominant and in a relationship with a submissive, but happens to get very sexually excited by being spanked.

That person may dominate their partner and say, "You will spank me now until I cum." We would say that person is dominant, but they are bottoming at that moment.

The submissive doing it would still consider themselves a submissive. They are a submissive who is topping for you, and we call that kind of situation service topping, meaning someone who is often playing the submissive role is topping because they have been told to do so.

There was a time long ago when the term *switch* had a negative connotation. It was said that a switch was someone who *couldn't make up their mind* about being dominant or submissive. Not to open up an even bigger can of worms, let's just say that most people today find that downright silly and extremely limiting. I would say that a majority of people starting out in the scene today identify as a switch or are at least interested in trying *both sides of the fence.*

More and more people are just having fun with BDSM and don't feel they need to take it so darn seriously. Many people just want to enjoy games of power with their partner. In this case, they really don't have to define themselves at all. Or maybe just call themselves *KINKY*, if they need to explain.

There are many more designations that mean different things to different people. As we mentioned before, often people will call someone a play partner. That usually denotes that that person is not quite as involved with their partner, it may just be a casual relationship, someone that you play with occasionally, someone that you play with all the time, but do not feel that they are quite your submissive, slave or bottom.

Another designation is what we call *collared*. To many people in our scene, a collar is very much like a wedding band, meaning that very often you will sign a contract with your partner, you will agree to terms, and you will begin your relationship when you are collared. You would then often be considered that person's slave.

Good luck getting a consistent description of what Collars and collaring means in the BDSM world. The differences can vary widely.

Some people go out to a party and have a quick fun evening together, and one or more of them will wear a collar. So for many people a collar is nothing more than a fashion statement.

When you see someone out at a party and they are wearing a collar, but are wearing it only as a fashion statement or just casually, should you tell those people: "You are not serious about this. You cannot wear that collar." NO! Wear five collars! Wear one as a ring in your nose!! Whatever makes you happy.

Often, people will decide to give someone a collar for the night. They might say, "You are going to be my play partner tonight so I am going to give you a collar to wear. That means that you are not going to play with anybody else. You are going to look after me tonight and attend to my needs." This is just another way. Not a better or worse way to approach collars, just different.

Some people that consider themselves dominant might wear a collar because in their mind they just like the way it looks. Again, if that works for you, then do it! However, as we said before, *usually* collaring tends to be more of a commitment in the BDSM world.

Also, the words master and slave can be confusing as well. Master is very similar to dominant and means the same thing in many different ways. However, master usually denotes that there is an even more serious and intense dynamic. The difference between a slave and a submissive is merely a mindset and you should use whatever terms feel right to you.

It is common that you might classify yourself as someone's master, dominant, and top and just have three different terms you can use where and when it suits you. The words are there to help us, not hinder us. And if you would like to be someone's slave a day after you meet, and you both think that works, there is no reason not to do that.

Again, every relationship is different. Sometimes this person may just be your dominant, sometimes they are your boyfriend, girlfriend, husband or wife as well. There is no standard for this. Just make sure to communicate and negotiate with your partner and be very clear about where you are in their life. Are you the girlfriend? Are you the boyfriend? Are you just the slave? Are you just the play partner? Are you a play partner who is a big part of this person's life or someone who you just play with once in a while? Make sure you discuss this with your partner.

Becoming the dominant

There is often a transformation that occurs when one steps into their dominant role. This is something that is very common that you may very well see with your partner, especially if they are more experienced. You can actually watch this person go from your equal, from your partner, to your dominant right before your eyes. This is how it should be if you are in a committed relationship with somebody and you wish to have a power dynamic. That person should be your equal one minute, and then when playtime starts, they should become that dominant in front of you. For some it might be imperceptible, for others it could be quite obvious and an extreme change. Regardless of which works for you, just remember when playtime starts, it is the time for you to be in character and become that person you wish to be.

Defining and Reinventing Yourself

As we said before, the TES creed states that we have the right to define ourselves, and that is a big part of what the BDSM scene is about.

Finding the dominant or submissive in you can be a complete renaissance of the soul, a new beginning, a new identity; It is very common to create a whole new name for your persona. If you are going to play outside of the confines of your home, this is also a good idea for safety. It is also completely normal to just go by your real name, but if you are not completely open with the world about your kink, then you may want to consider an alias when dealing with people online or in public.

Often people take honorifics like master so and so or slave so and so, sir, ma'am, etc. People often use sir and ma'am as signs of respect. Usually you will do okay using these respective titles if you want to show respect, but do not know how to address someone. The very best way is to simply ask.

People respond well to simple questions like, "It is very nice to meet you. May I ask you how you wish to be addressed?" This shows class and consideration, a big part of what we do.

Confidence

There is no one way to look as a dominant; it is whatever works for you. I have seen some of the most influential dominants look like the least imposing people possible and others look like the scariest bikers you've ever met.

That is because being a dominant has nothing to do with what you wear, it has to do with who you are.

Confidence is probably the single most important trait that a good dominant can have. This is the main thing that most submissives are looking for in a partner. Sometimes, being confident is easier said than done as we often derive confidence from our experience. As I often say:

Being new and being a dominant are cruelly in opposition of one another.

Being a dominant in the scene can be tough. I say this because when a dominant is new, they usually feel they must act like they know everything. After all, who would want to play with them if they do not know what they are doing? The truth is, there is nothing *worse* you can do.

Don't be the person who thinks, "Well, I am a dominant, so I guess the way to show that to people is to be really pushy and aloof, to lie about my experience and knowledge because I don't want to be found out."

The drive to be this way is rooted in our own insecurities that we hold inside us as dominants.

A real dominant wants to grow, they want to be better dominants and people.

I always say, as a coach, I want people to seek truth. I want them let go of their fears and find their integrity. When you stop growing, you start dying.

For me, I want to grow as a person. I want to be more in control of myself so that I am more deserving of the control I have of my partner. I feel that BDSM has been my medium to grow as person, to be more confident and a better human being.

There are dominants I met in the beginning of my journey who are still the same 20 years later; they are scared to be better. Usually, they are the ones that are the most clueless because they do not seem to want to grow as people.

Stagnation can be dangerous because when you have that kind of mentality and you have a new toy, you are going to lie to yourself and say "Hey, I know everything about this."

That is how people go 10 or twenty years and never improve because they are so busy telling everyone that they know everything, they certainly can never be caught dead learning anything.

Use BDSM to have a great time, but also use it as a great medium to grow as a person, together as a couple or separately as people. Think of it as this really hot, kinky self-help project.

The secret to being a dominant is developing QUIET CONFIDENCE.

To just be yourself. To wear what you want, be who you want to be and not feel pressured into any preconceived notion of what a dominant should be.

You need to realize that you DO NOT have to know everything on day one and it's totally normal to be nervous. Be polite, and affable instead of rude and aloof. Admit when you don't know something and show that you are interested in learning about it, don't lie and pretend you already do.

The reality is being dominant is NOT about how many toys you know how to use or how many people you know or how cool you can pretend to be. Luckily for you:

These things mean very little compared to simply being comfortable in your own skin. Take your time, and NEVER demand respect. Earn it instead.

If you have a hand and a brain, you can be a dominant. It's all in your head. If you *feel* like you are dominant, then you *are* dominant. And you don't have to prove that to anyone. Just know that you are.

Even the newest dominant is a great dominant for someone out there. Maybe not for everybody, but you are the perfect dominant for somebody out there even if you know very little. This can certainly be easier said than done. It will be difficult sometimes, but:

Trying your best to be humble and self-confident is the true key to success as a dominant. After all, if you can't be in control of yourself, what business do you have being in control of someone else?

Are you out to the world?

Often, I hear people ask

Does your family know?

I find that a bit baffling. Does *your* family know about your sex life? It seems for some reason that we, as people in the BDSM scene, are expected to share the intimate details of our sex life with our family, where vanilla people are not.

Quite frankly, it is really none of anybody's business what type of sex life you have, whether it is the most pure vanilla, monogamous, married sex or whether it is the crazy hanging from the chandelier with 12 people kind. This is really nothing that Grandma Joan needs to know.

If you have a tremendously open relationship with your mom or dad or brothers and sisters, it is also fine to let them know about your interest, but not necessarily from the sexual aspect, just from the social aspect.

However, if you are just a couple being kinky in the bedroom, then, really, there is no reason to be talking to your family about your sex life.

Do your friends know?

Once again, say whatever you wish to whomever you wish, but it is really none of their business that you have a dominant or your boyfriend owns five floggers and two whips. This is a private personal thing between you and your partner. That said, It is very difficult to have no one to speak to about all of the things you'll be experiencing. This is why it is a great idea to connect with others in the lifestyle. One way to do this is to have an account on *www.fetlife.com*, as I mentioned before.

If you are in a relationship with someone and just practicing BDSM privately, this is a great way for you to find some new friends who you can talk to about your interest without having to venture out into the world or taking the risk about telling a vanilla friend.

If you are interested in becoming part of the scene, then your local group is a great place to meet people and talk. The worst thing is to isolate yourself, especially if you have a lot of questions.

Again, if you are just having a little spanking on the butt and then having sex with your partner, you may really have nothing to share, and that is fine too. But when you do have a question, when you do need support, it is important to have a group or people that you can turn to, and FetLife.com is one great way to find some people like that, whether you want to venture out into the world or not.

Your inner demon – physicality/socialization

Hopefully, you were socialized not to use your physicality in a negative way as a child. Men don't hit women, and women are not supposed to ever kick a man in his balls. However metaphorical, this is exactly what we do in BDSM. We play around with the concept of *wrong*. Some things we do seem more socially acceptable than others. A simple spanking seems much less scary to many than pushing someone up against a wall by the throat or slapping them in the face.

It can take someone a long time to permit themselves to do the scarier things. Do not be surprised, when you start playing if you find it very difficult to do some of the things your partner wants to do.

After all, if you are in a loving relationship with someone and they are your primary partner, this is someone that you love and cherish and hopefully have a great relationship with, sometimes it is very difficult to turn around and hurt that person even if that is what they beg you for. Do not be put off by this. Do not be ashamed. This is how you are socialized, and it is a darn good thing you are.

It is absolutely not right to hit a woman or a man for that matter. It is absolutely not right for a woman to kick a man in the balls. These are things that we are socialized to not do and for good reason. You are merely displaying signs of your humanity when you have a trouble fulfilling some of these wants and desires.

This is very natural, and may or may not pass for you. Some people will never be comfortable doing some acts that their partner would like them to do. When this happens, you can often still provide these fantasies for your partner by doing them verbally.

For example, if your partner has a fantasy of being overwhelmed physically and in your mind, you feel you can never do something like that. This is fine, but does not mean that you cannot whisper to her about it in her ear as you are having sex.

So, remember, when something is too overwhelming for you to physically do, it is not necessarily too overwhelming to talk about or to fantasize about or to talk about while you having sex or masturbating.

Exploring primal feelings

Letting the inner demon out of its bag can be very difficult, even scary for most people, but tapping into primal feelings can actually be extremely exciting, and something that can be very liberating when you allow yourself to go there.

We are really all just animals with many animal instincts. Things like biting, hair pulling, and other dominant displays can be extremely liberating when they are consensual and we allow ourselves to feel comfortable with doing so.

Once again, the most important thing is to use communication. If you are feeling a bit nervous about grabbing your lover by the hair or biting them very hard, this is something to talk about.

When you are not playing, you may bring that up to them and say:

"Sometimes I feel like biting you, sometimes I feel like pulling your hair. How do you feel about that?"

You may be shocked to find that your partner is very excited by this. Even if they are not, this does not mean that you absolutely cannot do it because they may very well still give you permission, but are just letting you know that it is not something that they are interested in or understand about themselves.

Remember, there is a huge difference between someone thinking that they are interested in something in a generic way, as opposed to someone being interested in something because you are interested in it.

This is an important concept. You feel submissive or dominant with someone very often because of that person, because that is what that person or how that person makes you feel.

So while somebody may say, "eww, I do not like that at all. Biting is disgusting." That may be their feeling just in an everyday vanilla sense, but when they are in the throes of passion and in the middle of playing, doing BDSM activities, when they are bitten all of a sudden it is a whole different ball game, and may feel very, very exciting even though they had no thoughts that that would be the case.

Sometimes when we are in a vanilla headspace, we can imagine the things that would turn us on when we are in the middle of playing, but not always.

Do not be alarmed if your partner says they do not connect to the things that you want to do because as long as they don't tell you that it is off the table or revoke permission or remove consent for it, you can try it and see how it goes in the middle of your playtime. You will often be pleasantly surprised to find that, if it makes you hot and is something you want to do, in the right headspace, your partner will go along for the ride with you even if it is something they don't necessarily connect to as much as you do. Sometimes they might even develop quite an interest in it themselves.

The best way to introduce something like this is SLOWLY and a little at a time. If a partner allows you to try things on them that they don't think they will like, you should take that as a real sign of trust and affection and pay that back by gently introducing whatever activity we are talking about.

If you like to bite hard, bite a little less hard the first few times... you can work up to the heavy stuff as you move on. Want to slap someone in the face and they aren't sure about it? Try just tapping them the first time.

Face slapping happens to be a VERY intense thing for many people as they may have been disciplined that way. You'll find that just tapping certain people in the face can bring very intense reactions. This is the same for very many activities. So be careful.

Remember, we are playing a contact sport both physically and mentally, so take your time and always be observant of what is going on and communicate with your partner before, after and even during, if your style allows.

PAIN & PUNISHMENT

One of the questions that I am often asked is does BDSM have to hurt? And the answer is *absolutely not*, but it can be an awful lot of fun! There are so many different ways that you can play without pain. There is mental play, which we will discuss in a different chapter, where you are doing various things that are only in the mind.

There is mimicking heavier play with lighter implements, which many people do. You will see people using a fur flogger, for example, instead of a heavy leather flogger, and reenacting all the same things that someone would do with a traditional pain scene but with very light sensual touches. This is a very common way to play without pain.

There are also many people who are interested in roleplaying, where you are acting out various fantasies.

These are just a few examples of ways that you can play without pain involved. BDSM is such a creative sport, I am sure you can think of many different ways that you might be able to exchange power and play without pain.

However, many people in the scene do enjoy pain or play with pain and I usually see three different dynamics.

One is pain for the sake of pleasure. This is where a partner enjoys pain, and the partner will engage in some sort of role play perhaps or sometimes not, but they will give the partner pain so that they derive pleasure out of it. It may be in a role play where the opposite is being said and it may appear like the bottom is hating it, but really pleasure is the goal for this kind of situation.

The next is for punishment, especially for those of you that have a partner who does not like pain. As a matter of fact, you may have a partner who would be absolutely mortified to disappoint you enough that they would need to be punished. In this case, it's very much like a child and parent relationship, where the partner does as they are told, and if they do not do as they are told then they are punished with pain and other possible punishments.

Punishment is also used for discipline. Some people enjoy a dynamic where pain is used to reinforce various rules very much like a parent-child relationship or in the military world.

While corporal punishment is not extensively used in the military, there is quite a bit of emotional pain given when rules are not followed, and pain is given in a form of various calisthenics and other military punishments. The reenactment of a military-type atmosphere is very common for some.

The third would be kind of combination of the first two, which would be where you are playing around with punishment for pleasure.

A good example of that is a form of play called bratting. In this dynamic, one partner will misbehave on purpose until their partner punishes them.

The community is quite divided in this respect. For many people, this is a core dynamic. It is very popular for people who are interested in spanking because the dynamic is be bad, be bad, be bad, and then be spanked for being bad. Very much as a child would be spanked for being bad.

However, there are other people who find this dynamic appalling because they feel that, as my good friend Flagg once said:

> *"I do not need a reason to hurt you. I'll hurt you because I want to hurt you."*

Bratting can also be seen as, what people call, *topping from the bottom*. Although this may be a slight misuse of how the words top and bottom are usually used, what is being pointed out is that the submissive is actually leading the scene and topping by getting what they want from the dominant.

In other words, if a submissive is bratty to their dominant and keeps doing it until the dominant reacts, then some feel that this would a form of topping. Topping from the bottom is a phrase used to point by many to explain this activity.

The reason some people do not like topping from the bottom is because they feel it's manipulative. If you are a dominant and love to be in control, then you may very well not like your submissive bratting you into taking action.

However, if you are purely a sadist who enjoys giving pain and your partner enjoys receiving pain, then topping from the bottom does not have the same negative connotation. It is merely a dynamic where you are asking for pain in a roleplaying way.

So, why do we like pain?

Well, first of all, pain is sexually arousing for many people. Although the medical community is divided on why that may be, studies have shown that pain can have an almost antidepressant-type quality to it which is due to the various endorphins and chemicals in our brain that are released when we are in pain. There have also been studies that have shown that negative emotions subside when the body is under physical pain.

We should make a distinction that there are different kinds of pain, and as we noted above, depending on whether or not you are receiving pain as a punishment or for pleasure will definitely change the way you feel about the pain.

For the person above who is mortified by being bad and is being punished, punishment will not necessarily feel like good pain to them because of all the negative emotions that are associated with it.

Whereas pain for pleasure is a completely different mindset, and even though you may be roleplaying to the contrary, it is an enjoyable feeling of pain.

The very same person given the very same pain with the very same implement can be received completely differently depending on their mindset as to whether they have disappointed their dominant or whether the pain was being given to them in a pleasurable way.

Are we all sadists?

Not all dominants are sadists. Many have only a secondary or no interest at all in pain. They are interested in reactions or in giving their bottom pleasure, often both.

For many people, pain is more of a means to an end. They know their partner enjoys it, so they give it to them. If they, for one moment, thought that their partner was not enjoying it, they would immediately stop, as they see a major difference between the two. One is abusive pain. The other is pleasurable pain.

Many people are what I call *reaction junkies*. Reaction junkies are people who enjoy their partners' reactions. I believe it to be a deep internal need that many people must affect their surroundings, and it is not surprising that it would be part of their sexual identity as well.

For some people, begging, suffering, laughing, crying, it does not really matter, they just love getting an intense reaction from their partner. These type of people would be aghast if they hurt their partner in a way they did not mean to hurt them because pain is not the real objective. The reaction is.

Also, there are people who do not enjoy inflicting pain at all because they are what you call a service top. Basically, their partner enjoys pain, their partner is a masochist. They are not a sadist, but they want to give their partner pleasure.

This often will be the case where there may be two submissives in a relationship together. When the one gives the other one pain, it is done purely as a service top, not as a dominant, meaning they derive no pleasure out of the actual act of giving pain and might even dislike it, but it is something they do for their partner as requested, and this aspect gives them pleasure.

Sociopaths

I am often asked if pure sadists truly exist in BDSM that are not sociopaths. My answer is, I do not know.

I have met seemingly well-adjusted people who call themselves sadists, but there always seem to me to be more to their relationship than just pure sadism. I think we are dealing with semantics and what your definition of a sadist is. I have also met some very dark people who consider themselves sadists that I would term sociopaths.

The concept of sociopathy and how it manifests in the BDSM scene is a long conversation for a different book, but for the sake of what we are trying to learn in this book, I would just say: If your partner is interested purely in hurting you with absolutely no dynamic of pleasure or any type of connection, then you probably want to seriously consider if this is a relationship for you.

The keyword is connection.

Just because someone is interested in being a sadist does not make them a bad person.

But if they want to be a sadist and have absolutely no connection to you, your wellbeing, and your pleasure, then there is a good chance you are dealing with a sociopath.

There is a huge difference between playing with power, playing with various concepts that make us aroused, and having an illness that prevents us from feeling anything.

Bruises and marks

Sometimes when people enjoy pain, they also enjoy bruises. This may be surprising to some, but really, when explained, it makes a lot of sense.

Most people who enjoy bruising see it almost as a trophy or remembrance. They may touch their bruises during the day to remind themselves of the playtime they had the night before. They may look at the bruises in the mirror to remember what happened. Similar to how a vanilla person might view a hickey.

To those people, bruises are basically sexy reminders of the fun time they had. That said, many people will never play to that intensity, nor should they. They will never have a bruise. They will never have a mark. And that's ok too. Again, this is one of those things that is completely up to you and what you like.

Pain is relative

What is heavy to one person is light to someone else and vice versa. You need to be very careful about how you inflect pain on someone else and to not assume that the person's pain tolerance is similar to yours or whoever you may have played with before. People's pain also changes from day to day, month to month, or week to week.

One of the things about pain play is that it can bring catharsis. Catharsis can be defined as a purification or purge. This is another very popular reason people enjoy pain play. For some people, intense pain will cause catharsis, where huge amounts of stress and negative energy will leave the body during this time. Many people feel pain can be a purification and bring about healing.

People have used pain to reach catharsis and transcend since the dawn of time. There are many reports of pain being used in various religious and spiritual ceremonies. One might picture a Native American hanging by chest hooks looking into the sky or worshipers flogging their backs as they walk to an Easter church service in the Philippines.

Crying

Which brings us to crying. Crying is a very different experience for different people. But, often, it is the end of a cathartic scene. It is important to make sure you communicate with your partner so you know the difference between good crying and bad crying.

Some people find it very difficult to watch the person they love or, at the very least, care for, cry. But, for some, this is the actual goal of their play. For many, a good scene is one with prolonged intense pain that brings catharsis and ends with deep sobbing and emotional purging.

It is perfectly understandable if the dominant has a problem dealing with watching their partner cry. All dominants must realize that they have limits as well, but especially male dominants. Men are socialized to *never hit a women*, and so it is understandable that when engaging in that very act, even consensually, it could bring up deep feelings of shame and self-loathing.

It is often very hard for a new dominant to deal with this intensity. Hence, one should not feel funny about making crying or anything else for that matter, a limit for the dominant.

In this case, intense cathartic play might not be possible for the partners or at least catharsis that ends in crying. This does not mean that the dominant will never be able to deal with this, but there is going be a lot of communication needed, a lot of talking and a lot of reassurance before the dominant will feel okay with doing that.

Also, a lot of aftercare is needed after such a scene so that all parties can feel better about themselves and not feel guilty.

Shame is a big part of BDSM, and when we do heavy play, there can be shame felt on both sides. The partner receiving the pain may feel ashamed that they enjoy such a taboo act the dominant or top may feel ashamed that they would do such a thing.

TOYS & ACTIVITIES

When you first start playing in the scene, your hand and your brain will be your first toys

Almost everybody eventually wants to learn how to use all those great toys that they see everyone playing with and do all the cool things they see people doing.

In this chapter, we are going to discuss some you may want to get involved with, some you may not, and advice on how to play with them safely.

First, it is a great idea to try a toy on yourself. Having empathy and understanding how a toy might feel is a big help. Remember, everybody experiences pain differently. So, just because it feels pretty comfortable to you at a certain intensity does not mean that it will feel that way to someone else. However, it's still good for you to at least get an idea of how intense a toy is.

You can hit your arm or the side of your leg with a toy or, if you are using a flogger, flog yourself on your back. Get a good feel for the toy before you use it on other people.

One of the most important things is to warm up. No matter what toy you use, you do not want to just walk over and start whaling away on somebody. Whaling away on somebody is a good way for someone to get hurt.

You should always be in control of your toy. I know sometimes when you are new, you will be nervous, and it might be your first instinct to just try to hit very hard.

Fight that instinct. That is the exact opposite of what you want to do.

You should almost always start by hitting your partner softly. This is a great way for you to warm them up and warm yourself up as well! If you are using, let's say, a crop in your hand, you can slowly touch different parts on your partner's body and feel how that crop reacts as you connect with it. It will make your eye-hand coordination much better because you are starting off very slow and easy.

Do not forget that you want to communicate with your partner about how a toy feels. When you first start playing with a toy, you really want to get some feedback.

That means that, although you can do some light roleplaying, you'll only want to do the kind that allows you to talk to your partner about their experience. Yes, you can still be sexy and commanding if you wish, but the first time, it's really better to just be on a fact finding mission and play in a power neutral way with each other.

Take a new toy and hit your partner with it, then ask them how it feels. Get feedback and try it again. This is a wonderful way to try out a toy, and if you are new, I strongly suggest this be the only the way that you should start out.

I've separated some toys and activities into three different low, medium, and high-risk sections.

Low risk

This, meaning that, obviously, the lower risks are easier to use and have less risk physically and mentally to your partner.

Any toy used incorrectly, in the wrong spot or in an extreme way can take it from a low-risk toy to a high-risk toy.

Our first low-risk activity is a simple blindfold.

Taking away one of your partner's senses is a great way to start out a scene. When you put that blindfold on for the first time, all kinds of interesting things happen. First, your partner realizes instantly that they are dependent on you and that they need to have a certain level of trust to allow it to happen.

Also when you take away someone's senses, everything intensifies. Your partner will await your next move with an intensity that you've never before seen. Just blindfolding someone and stepping back and watching them for a few minutes can be a scene in itself!

Next is spanking.

Spanking is probably the most common activity to start with. It is the easiest for most people because you are not using a toy, rather only your hand.

A spanking is something that can be very, very personal and intimate between two parties because you are hitting someone with your hand and not a toy.

If you are hitting somebody on the butt and upper thigh area where most people like to be spanked, cup your hand a bit while you are doing the spanking so that it actually fits the person's anatomy when you hit it and you will get a better feel.

Remember, do not go too hard too fast. Start very lightly. Maybe run your fingers and tease the person all over before you start spanking. That can feel wonderful, and then the spanking after can be quite a different feeling.

Riding Crops are another low-risk activity.

The shorter ones with the firmer tips are usually called bats. But a crop or a bat is another toy that is very firm and easy to use.

Be very careful when you use this toy. Unless you are trying to turn it into a high intensity toy, do not hit the person with the rod. Only hit the person with the tip. Use the tip and hit the person where you want to put the sensation. Since most crops are very firm and have a small tip at the end, they are very easy to control. You can use one very, very lightly or very, very hard.

The next is paddling.

You can use many different items for a paddle, and the sky is the limit. There certainly are lovely leather and wood paddles that you can purchase, but you could find almost anything around the house. A wooden spoon, a hairbrush, a book a piece of wood, etc.

I am including in here with paddling, things like rulers and anything firm and long. A paddle is another toy that is easy to use because it is a firm object. When you hold it in your hand, it will not move around and will impact exactly where you want it.

However, you need to be mindful when using longer paddles or longer toys in general. Longer toys can cause what we call wrapping, which is often unpleasant for the submissive or the bottom. We'll talk more about wrapping in a few pages

You need to remember that depending on the angle you use, the entire paddle may be striking the person. So, be very careful. Either only use the tip of the paddle and watch that, or, if you are using the entire paddle, focus on the surface where the paddle is landing. Remember to make sure you are hitting a safe spot on the body (take a look at our safety chapter for more information on this).

Use extremes to your advantage. Hitting with a hard item then doing something very light and tender with your fingers can be lovely, and the difference between the two is what makes the highs higher and the lows lower. So the more you touch and tingle, the more that the heavier playing will register.

Tickling is an interesting form of play.

Teasing and tickling is another very low-risk, fun, and sensual way to play. Running your fingers over somebody's body is highly underrated. When you go for a massage, often the masseuse with run their fingers lightly all over your body and it is truly one of the best feelings you can have.

Some people enjoy being tickled and others will tear your heart out if you even threaten it. Tickling is a great low-risk activity that you can do to get someone to react rather extremely to you without hurting them physically.

Tickling is also a good example of how some activities that seem very innocent can be perceived as intense by certain partners. Many people were tormented as children with tickling, so if you tie those people up and tickle them; some will enjoy it like any other form of BDSM, but others will have a very bad experience.

This is true of all BDSM activities so never forget how important communication and negotiation is for *all* activities, not just the ones that you *think* it would be needed for.

Gags

Are another way of taking away one of your partner's senses, like a blindfold does. Be careful with gags, some people don't do well having something in their mouth and, appropriately enough, their *gag* reflex will kick in. Also, once someone has a gag in their mouth they can no longer give you their safeword orally and you'll have to figure out something to keep the scene consensual. Putting something in their hand to drop or telling them to grunt three times are two ideas that can stand in for a regular safeword.

There are many ways to do bondage.

You can use rope. You can use wraps like an ace bandage or vet wrap. You can do mummification with saran or pallet wrap. You can put people in restraints and various different cuffs.

Most of these are pretty safe, but you have to be careful of a few things.

First is cutting off the blood flow to a part of the body. If, for example, you use rope, be mindful that rope is notorious for cutting blood flow off. Be very careful. If someone's hands or extremities start to get cold or change color, they need to be untied and the blood needs to be let back into that part of the body. So, be very careful about keeping good blood flow, and communicate with your partner and let them know that you want to know if their arms start to go to sleep or their wrists and hands start to fall asleep. This is important information that you need to know.

If you are going to use rope:

You need to own safety scissors.

Safety scissors are a very inexpensive item, usually under five dollars. They are indispensible for safe bondage. Don't worry about cutting the rope, no matter how expensive. No rope is worth harming your partner. You need to be able to get them out quickly, very quickly. Actually, if you are going to do any kind of bondage, you should have safety scissors. Regardless of what you use for restraint, there is the possibility that it won't come off fast enough and will need to be cut off.

The third thing you have to worry about is balance. Be very careful when you tie somebody up. If you tie them standing up, they can fall right over. Regardless of how you tie them, you still need to always watch them. When bound, your partner cannot stop themselves from falling like they would if they had their arms or legs free, so stay vigilant.

Another important thing is to never leave a person in bondage unsupervised. You must always be able to see your partner when they are in bondage. Bad things could happen if you walk away and they have no one there to help them if they need it. You can create an illusion of you going away by blindfolding your partner and pretending to open and close the door, but -

Do not leave your partner unsupervised when they are in bondage. Ever.

Saran wrap can be a lot of fun, and we all have some right in the kitchen. Any type will do, but I suggest you get the largest roll you can find at the grocery store. You can start at the ankles and wrap up the body. Be careful that the ankle bones aren't touching and rubbing together as that can be painful. Try to offset them a bit. To start off, wrap a few times around one of the ankles so there is a bit of a cushion between them. Also, be careful as you get up to the face; do not cover your partner's mouth and nose. Saran wrap can actually get tighter, so if you wrap around the person's chest, have them take a deep breath in as you are wrapping. That will leave them enough room to breathe once the wrap is on.

After the wrap is on the body, use a pair of safety scissors to cut out special spots, like the breasts, and other private areas you'd like to get to. Feel free to add more saran wrap to complete your masterpiece as you see fit.

Now we move on to medium-risk activities...

One would be clothespins and clamps.

If you go to your local grocery store or to your Home Depot, you will find clothespins in abundance.

There are all different types of clothespins. The reason that we put this in medium-risk is because clothespins vary greatly in intensity and you need to be very aware of that as you put them on the body. Also clothespins hurt MUCH worse coming off then going on. Remember that the longer you leave them on, the longer you are cutting off the blood flow and the more painful it will be when you take them off and restore the flow.

You can get wooden clothespins of varying intensity. Some are very light and soft, and don't really put much pressure on at all. Others are heavier and give a good clamp. There are plastic clothespins, which can be very different in intensity and there are different clamps and clips that act like clothespins. Some of those can be very, very high intensity.

So, you have to be careful. Generally, wooden clothespins should not be more than medium intensity. Once you get into plastic or anything else, you are dealing with something that could be extremely high intensity.

Do not put clamps on somebody without trying them on yourself.

Remember, if you put them on your hand or your finger, that is not what it feels like to somebody when it is on their nipples or other sensitive areas. Remember, people's breast, nipple, and genital flesh are much more sensitive than your fingers.

Clothespins can be a lot of fun, and you can buy a whole bunch of them and put them in a whole bunch of different spots all over the body. They are inexpensive and can be found anywhere. I suggest that when you are done playing with them, you simply throw them away for cleanliness purposes. However, if you only play with one person, then keeping them and reusing them is really not a problem.

Next would be caning.

You would need to purchase a cane or use something that is long, straight, and sticklike. Canes are traditionally made of rattan wood, but you can buy ones made of plastic and different synthetic materials. You can buy them online and in many different places.

Caning is right in the middle between high-risk and low-risk and can become either pretty quickly. It can be low-risk because, again, a cane is a solid item that is easy to control. You can hit somebody with it and do it very lightly if you like. However, canes can be used with extreme intensity and have the potential to be very painful and easily cut the skin; it's up to you to be very careful how you use one.

When you use a cane, be very careful. Start very lightly and work up slowly. This is one implement that you have to be very concerned about wrapping, meaning that if you do not watch the end it is very possible for it to start whipping around the body and hit places you do not want to hit.

Aim the cane so that the tip is hitting a good spot on the body. If you are using it on someone's butt, don't let the end of the cane go further than the butt cheek itself because if you have it so that the middle of the cane is hitting the butt cheek, the tip of the cane will come around and hit the side of the person's body, which is not a pleasurable place to be hit.

Note: sting and thud are the two types of pain that people usually associate with toys. The thinner something is, the more stingy it usually feels. The thicker and more massive something is, the more thud it will cause.

A cane is at the high end of stingy. Some people love stingy, some people hate it. A paddle, although it is still stingy, is usually considered thuddy because there is so much more surface space that is hitting the body and spreading out the energy from the blow.

Floggers come in a multitude of styles

Flogging is another very popular type of play. A flogger is any kind of whip that has multiple tails and usually a rigid handle. Flogging can be very easy for some people, especially if they've participated in certain sports in the past or have good eye-hand coordination. However, others find flogging rather daunting.

Floggers vary from those that are very light and soft bunny fur all the way up to the heaviest and most intense rubbers and boot laces, and everything in between. When you are starting out, I would recommend a nice medium length, double elk flogger, which is thick, and fairly heavy, but still a soft and supple leather flogger.

I recommend you purchase them at www.detailstoys.com.

(For the sake of complete disclosure the writer of this book happens to be part owner of DetailsToys.com, but even if I wasn't, I'd still recommend this great lifestyle company that has been around for over 15 years.)

The next flogger that we usually recommend, if you wanted a second, would be a bull flogger. Bull is much heavier, and sometimes people want to feel a heavier feeling on their body. If you have a medium double elk and a single medium bull, those two floggers will get you most of the sensations you are looking for.

Now, of course, there are literally endless combinations of floggers that you can purchase from a place like detailstoys.com. You can get the super soft fur floggers, medium, but stingy, suede floggers, intense and thuddy buffalo floggers and extremely high end latigo or rubber floggers, just to name a few.

By all means, feel free to try them all, but when you are first starting out, a double elk medium and a single medium bull are the perfect starter set.

I am also going to teach you right now my fool proof method for safely using a flogger so you will never again feel nervous about using one with your partner.

Step one: take your flogger and swing (aka throw) it. Throw it at a wall, throw it at a pillow, throw it wherever you want, but throw it and get used to how it feels. I don't want you to worry about certain types of throws, just do whatever feels comfortable for you. Your only job when you are throwing is to make sure that you can get the very tips of the tails to go where you want them.

Once you feel pretty comfortable doing that, take your flogger in your hand and get behind you partner. Decide where you are going to hit, and swing your flogger

BUT miss on purpose.

Do not hit them. Stay a foot away from the spot you are trying to hit. As you are swinging your flogger and trying to hit them, just slowly move your body towards your partner. Just lean in a little bit, move your feet slightly, whatever you need to do, but just inch closer to the spot.

The idea is to develop a stroke that you can repeat over and over again, putting the tips where you want them. Do not worry about the rest of the flogger.

Again, we need to talk about wrapping. If you swing your flogger and try to aim the middle of the flogger for where you want, you are going to be hitting all kinds of places you did not want to hit.

Simply try to put the tips of your flogger on a safe part of your partner's body by doing that missing on purpose and then slowly leaning in to your target or moving your body closer technique. There is no need to be nervous. It is just like taking some practice cuts in the batting cage before you play baseball or shooting a few hoops before you start the game. You want to practice throwing it a little bit and feeling the toy in your hand.

By the way, if you would like to learn about floggers, I strongly recommend you go to *www.detailstoys.com* and buy the wonderful flogger DVD, "The Details of

Flogging." This flogging tutorial is 3.5 hours long and covers both the physical and mental sides of the scene. It offers you four of the top teachers in the scene and you may even recognize one of them (Not to ruin the surprise but it's me...you might recognize me).

Now, moving up to more high-risk activities...

Let's start with knives.

If you are new in the scene, you should not be using a knife for anything other than scaring somebody and you need to be extremely careful when you do it.

If you are going to put a sharp knife on your partner's body, be very careful. Remember, just the slightest movement could impale them and injure them severely. However, some people really enjoy being scared by knives and you may really want to use one.

One way to make it safer is to use a knife with a dull edge, which will make the toy less scary, but much safer. Regardless of which type you use, make sure you show this implement the respect it deserves. Again, when you are new, keep to using it as a fear toy and wait till you have more experience before you try anything more intense with it.

Then there is face slapping

Face slapping is an emotionally high-risk activity because, really, you are not going to usually hit somebody hard enough to cause a lot of physical damage. However, you can cause a lot of psychological damage.

One way to see if a partner has any interest in being slapped in the face would be to lightly put your hand on their cheek and just tap it a little bit and watch for the reaction. Of course, the very best way would be to have read their negotiation form or simply ask your partner how they feel about being slapped in the face. But if you are in the middle of a scene and you would like to try it out, just lightly tap their face. If they react very suddenly and pull away, it is probably nothing you want to do until you have had a good long conversation about it. In general, it is always better to first talk about something that has the opportunity for psychological trauma.

Consensual non-consent

Consensual non-consent is the act of playing around with the idea of ignoring consent. Of course this is a very slippery slope since BDSM is built on the foundation that there must be consent at all times. Luckily we have safewords that allow us to give our partner the illusion of non-consent.

It is very common for a partner to want to fight against you or simply have you ignore their pleas for mercy. Just be sure that you have a safeword in place so that the scene can stay consensual even though you are *pretending* it isn't.

WARNING: This can be one of the most traumatic ways you can play with your partner as you might be exploring rape contexts or other heinous acts within this fantasy context.

Do not, I repeat, do not play with consensual non-consent without speaking to your partner about it first.

It is far too traumatic for some people to take the chance. You need to discuss it; It does not necessarily have to be discussed the day you are going to try it, but you must verbally discuss it with your partner prior to engaging in consensual non-consent. Do not play around with it no matter how popular it seems without talking to your partner.

Another high-risk activity would be choking.

We've all heard about people who have died from restricting air intake.

Do not do play with choking lightly, your partner can die.

When you are new, I recommend you do not do any kind of choking or breath play unless you have negotiated it fully with your partner. I would also recommend not restricting your partner's airway by putting your hands around their neck.

Until you know what you are doing, you can severely injure somebody by trying to restrict their air at their neck. If you have negotiated it with your partner and you both still want to do breath play, the best way to do it is to use one hand to pinch the nose and another hand to cover the mouth.

Usually a person can get a little bit of air that way. It can still be very, very frightening and scary, but you take zero risk of crushing their trachea or hurting your partner's neck in any way.

That said, it can be very sexy to grab somebody by the neck and push them up against the wall or control them, but there is a major difference. When you control someone by the neck, you are not squeezing, you are merely holding them by the neck. Once you start squeezing, that is when you are looking for trouble. Do not squeeze the neck when you are new. There is too much risk involved. You do not want to end up in the newspapers tomorrow, as, unfortunately, some have over the years.

Get whipped into shape.

Whipping is something best left to people who are very interested in learning the art of whipping and want to practice it quite a bit. When I say whipping, I mean using a single-tail whip, for example a signal whip, a bullwhip or a snake whip. The signal whip is one of the most common whips used in the BDSM world, but is absolutely not for beginners. One errant hit from a single tail whip can cut someone's flesh and incur a trip to the hospital.

Do not ever swing a single tailed whip aimed at anyone unless you have many, many hours of experience using a whip and/or have taken classes to use them safely. Whip throwing is a fun activity, whip cracking is very fun too, but cracking and throwing on a human can be extremely dangerous.

I always tell people that unless you are really, really interested in learning and putting the time in to learn how to use singe-tails, there are other toys that are much easier to use, much cheaper to buy, and that require no breaking-in and much less education time.

Roleplaying

Roleplaying is a big part of what we do in the BDSM world. Unless you are a strict masochist or sadist, you are doing some form of role play when you are playing with your partner.

Basically, we are playing a grown up version of make believe. When role playing, we free ourselves of our normal boundaries, and find out some interesting new things about ourselves. Acting out your fantasies is an extremely healthy way to explore your sexual life in general and a really HOT part of BDSM.

There is absolutely nothing wrong with experimenting with different forms of sexual play, provided both partners are interested in it.

How do we find out if both partners are interested in it?

We ask! It's as simple as that, we negotiate, we talk, we fill out negotiation forms, and we do anything we possibly can to communicate.

For help with this type of communication, please visit the communication chapter in this book. One of your best role play friends is the negotiation form that we suggest there.

There are different types of role play. Sometimes we like to play serious, full-on characters, where we really try to be convincing and take on a different personality for a brief amount of time. Sometimes we just enjoy some fun, tongue-in-cheek type role play, like being the silly naughty doctor playfully examining his patient. Neither is right or better, they are just different types, and you might enjoy one style or both.

It's important to realize that even if you are doing something as simple as a spanking, you are taking on a role. Even if it's just you magnified. After all, you don't ordinarily go around spanking people in your regular life.

How to be a BETTER roleplayer

Roleplaying is actually exactly like being an actor.

The American Academy of Dramatic Arts in NYC taught me that

Acting is truthfully and spontaneously working off the behavior of others moment to moment under imaginary circumstances

So the thing to remember when we role play is the word PLAY. When you are a kid, you are a great actor, you have nothing to feel self-conscious about, you'll try anything. That's where we want to get to when we role play.

You want to be yourself, but under imaginary circumstances. You want to be in the moment, you want to have fun. You want to just go for it and throw caution to the wind, listen and react

Roleplay allows us to do things we would never ordinarily be able to do. For example, we might try being extremely outgoing if we are shy or vice versa. We could pretend we are a different age, social status, gender, etc.

Roleplay allows us to act out events we would never ordinarily condone. We might want to play out a consensual non-consent scene like a rape or kidnapping. We might want to inflict merciless torture on someone and have them beg for mercy.

We need to keep in mind that although we are in a fantasy world, real-world safety rules apply, even to a greater degree. Since a person is acting and letting themselves go, you really don't know when they are being serious and when they are acting. Safewords are a MUST when we role play.

Also, mental pain is even more possible while role-playing. You must be vigilant to watch out for this. For example, many of the topics that are most intriguing to play around with are some of the most taboo and have potential minefields attached to them.

You might want to do age play or daddy/girl/boy play or, as we mentioned before, consensual non-consent (rape) play. This is very common, but since anywhere from 25-50 percent of all people are molested at some point, in some way in their lifetime, there is a very good possibility that there may be some issues that could come up or a bad experience could happen.

Remember, when we indulge in this play we want to make sure we keep it safe, sane and consensual.

- Safe: meaning nothing that would cause permanent physical or mental damage.

- Sane: either one of you may very well not be in your right mind while you are playing and it's both your responsibilities to be ready to safeword and pause the scene if you are worried that this is happening.

- Consensual: meaning that you both consent to everything before and during the scene.

Structuring the Fantasy

When you are thinking of creating a fantasy, the first thing you need to do is fantasize. Start to dream of what you want to do. How will it happen? See it in your mind's eye.

Once you've thought it up, you can decide whether you want it to be a surprise or not. If it's not a surprise, then you want to talk about it with your partner. Get their feedback and have them do the same thing. Have them close their eyes and fantasize. What would make it sexy and hot for them? What would happen that would be exciting?

If the fantasy is going to be a surprise, then you want to at least talk to your partner enough about the fantasy that you know what are the things they will and won't do. What are their limits? Using the aforementioned negotiation form is a great way to help you do this. If you are the type of player that likes to take their partner by surprise, reading over a fully filled out negotiation form will let you know a lot about what your partner is okay with. Remember, however, that negotiation forms are just one part of the puzzle and are never a replacement for good ole' verbal communication. Set your boundaries with your partner and make sure you have an established safeword.

Remember, while usually being extremely fun and rewarding, this kind of play can go wrong quickly, so it's essential that you use safewords when you are role-playing! Then just let go and have fun. No one is watching, no one is judging, this is a time to play like a child and live out all the fantasies you've ever dreamed of.

Once you are done with the fantasy, take care of your partner and enjoy some time together or apart if that's what floats your boat. Later, you'll want to debrief with each other and talk about what went right, what went wrong, and how you enjoyed it. Do homework as outlined in my triangle of communication in the communication chapter of this book.

THE MENTAL SIDE

BDSM is a state of mind.

Submission is something that someone chooses to do consensually. Submission can't be taken, it must be freely given.

This is all done in the mind. This has nothing to do with hitting someone, spanking or any other physical form of play.

Remember, first, you must stimulate someone's mind before you can stimulate their body. When someone chooses to give you their submission, this should be looked at as a great honor. An honor that they feel you are worthy of their submission.

A Word About Integrity

Integrity is everything in BDSM. If you wish for somebody to submit to you mentally, they must truly believe you are worthy of that submission. They must trust you implicitly.

To be worthy, you must have integrity.

Your partner must respect you and believe that you are someone they wish to subjugate themselves to. Do not think for a minute that you can come in and physically compel someone to bend to your will.

That is a prisoner, not a willing participant.

I know many of you would like to do things the easy way and merely command someone to do what you want. Unfortunately, this is not what we are after in BDSM. That is what you are after in abuse.

This is where my comments in the beginning of the book about personal growth really come into play. As a dominant, you need to realize that you should always aspire to getting better. You need to be more trustworthy; you need to have more integrity; you need to grow as a person in order to be worthy of someone following you.

This is very much like in the vanilla world, where you may have a boss who is a jerk and does not do their job well, and you might never truly submit or go along with their program because they do not inspire you and your participation.

However, if you have a boss who is filled with energy, integrity, good humor or any of the other traits that make someone inspiring, it is often said that you would go to hell and back with that person.

If your partner feels submissive in general, then they will want you to be this person. They will be rooting for you. Having you be at your best makes them feel good about themselves.

This brings up yet another point of wanting your partner to be the best that they can be. Many dominants make the mistake that it's somehow a positive thing to put down someone else to make yourself feel better.

That is definitely something that you see in the BDSM world sometimes and it is very sad. You would think that a dominant would realize that the more powerful a person their partner is, the more that person has to give the dominant, and not the other way around.

Build up yourself, build up your partner. Together, you can have an extremely exciting sex life but also an extremely exciting life in general. Break out of those ruts and remember:

When you stop growing, you start dying.

Humiliation

Mental play is just as much of a form of BDSM as in the physical realm. All the same rules apply. You are completely equal outside of the bedroom or outside of the times that you agreed to play in.

One of the biggest forms of mental play is humiliation. It is important for people to realize that when we are talking about humiliation play, we are not talking about making somebody feel bad about themselves or ripping or tearing somebody down. That is usually abusive. That is not what we are doing.

A good example of tearing someone down would be calling an overweight partner fat, it would probably be devastating to your partner for you to humiliate them by speaking to them in that way. Although it is intense, and will certainly get a reaction, it is a little bit too close to home and will probably take your partner right out of headspace and feel terrible about themselves.

Often when people answer whether or not they are interested in humiliation on their negotiation forms, they will say no but not realize what you mean.

There is huge difference between telling somebody that they are terrible, useless, and worthless, than telling them that they are *your* little worthless or *your* little useless girl/boy.

It's subtle, but there is a major difference in how you mean it and how you say it. If you are saying it to your partner purely because you feel that they really are useless or you feel that they are fat or you feel that there is something else that you have an issue with, you need to deal with it away from BDSM.

> *BDSM is not a convenient way for you to air your grievances with a partner who won't defend themselves because they are in a submissive head space.*

BDSM is a way to play around with taboo subjects and have a good time. Successful humiliation play is all about how you mean it. You can say the meanest thing to someone and sound very convincing, but if you are doing it because you are connected to your partner and you know it makes them excited to hear, then it's completely different than saying it in a soul crushing way.

Playing around with intense emotions is a mine field and you need to be very careful how you navigate it. Even when you do everything right, there will still be times where you might go too far and your partner may feel bad. If this happens to you, remember that the way to make it all better is through communication. Make sure your partner knows that you were just trying to role play and it didn't go quite the way you planned.

Playing with Wrong

What is it about doing things that are wrong that is so darn appealing? What is it that is so exciting about playing around with taboo subjects, guilt and shame?

What I found over the years is that many of us who are interested in the scene fall into the reaction junkie category. We enjoy any type of reaction, any outward expression like a laugh, cry, scream, beg, plead, and even inward expressions, shame, guild, anger, affection, or revulsion.

I believe that on a base level, human beings have a need to affect and be affected by other people. It is well-documented that humans need companionship, and my feeling is that through reactions we somehow fill this need on a deep level.

Like any fetish, there is no exact reason why we chose to connect on this level. But nonetheless, I believe this is all about connection between partners. "You poke me, I say ouch." It is certainly a strange way to connect, but a connection, nonetheless, and one highly favored by the BDSM community.

Many of us reaction junkies enjoy reactions away from the scene as well. I have to thank my wife and my other two partners for putting up with me all these years as I do not like to just push buttons in the scene, but on a day-to-day basis.

For example, most women, my wife and partners included, are not big fans of scatological humor. You can be assured that I will break out every poop joke and poop song parody that could ever be created at the smallest provocation.

I don't think that I even do it on purpose. It is literally just a deep need for me. I find myself doing it constantly with friends and especially play partners. I just love reactions. And as I said, I believe it is a form of connection.

When I was in high school and first figuring out that I was kinky, one of my big fetishes was tickling. I was not interested in the *koochie koochie koo* type cute tickling. For me, it was all about watching people react strongly to something I was doing.

As I grew and learned more about something called BDSM, I realized that it was not just tickling that interested me, but it was intense reactions that was my true interest. From there, my interest in BDSM grew, and although tickling remains a core fetish of mine, it was sort of a gateway fetish that helped me understand what it was I really wanted.

One of my favorite quotes is, "I want to know everything about you so I can liberally use it against you." This quote sort of sums up how reaction junkies feel. We want to know everything possible about you so we can turn it into one of the paints in our paint box, and help use it to create our art, which is what we call a scene.

So, how do we find out what is "wrong?" It can be a big turn on actually finding out all this information that you want to get. I love the puzzle aspect of this and the creative element. As you already learned, one very good way to find out what is "wrong" is using my triangle of communication, which includes clear and consistent verbal communication, negotiation forms, and homework.

Besides that, observation is one of the biggest ways to find out what is *wrong*. We want to be in relentless pursuit of information.

My hobby is constantly looking for nuggets that I can use in a future play scene. The idea is to truly soak up as much information as you can about your partner. This does not have to be obvious sexual things, but mundane day-to-day things can become huge important bits of information at some point in the future.

We must remember that playing around with wrong is edgeplay. We are pushing mental limits. Obviously, teasing someone a bit about something is on the low end of the edgeplay, but when we get into playing with very, very deep shameful and other wrong feelings, we are certainly pushing the limits and the edges to someone's capacity.

We must remember to always have a safeword in place between you and your partner to be able to keep things consensual. This is also a time where you need to be very observant of your partner and their limits as many people may not be able to safeword because they are feeling deep emotions, such as shame and guilt.

Start slowly and the rest will come naturally. Your skills of observation and rationalization will be tested, and you will learn how not to go too far. It is very important that after you do scenes that deal with humiliation and other taboo topics, you check in and find out from your partner through verbal communication and homework how they felt about the playtime. I am going to share with you a homework entry I once received that sums things up nicely. It might actually seem very tame to you, but for this person, it was very intense.

Somehow, on Saturday he got me to confess, that watching him do a scene with another partner and helping him do stuff to her would turn me on. What am I crazy? I guess you just hate to admit that something that you don't like on one level at the same time turns you on too. It SUCKS! You feel as if your body is betraying what your mind says about something. Or more realistically, it's not even what your mind says, but your body is betraying everything you were brought up to believe, your value system, the ideals that you were taught growing up.

There are many types of play that can evoke intense reactions, things that would be considered *playing with wrong*.

Some of the more intense things could be rape, incest, molestation, race, religion, etc. Your question right now might be:

"Why would we want to do this?"

"Why would we want to play around with such taboo subjects?" "I'm a good person. I would never do that."

It's very important to point out that you should NOT do it if makes you uncomfortable. There is no reason you have to do it. But strong powerful feelings have the potential for strong powerful excitement. Playing with this kind of feeling is amazingly powerful. Shame, guilt, betrayal, morals, ethics, greed, these are all feelings that are extremely intense and bring about extreme excitement.

Why this happens? I don't know, but I can only tell you that it is very true that the more intense you go mentally, most of the time, the more intense you feel sexually.

It is very important that you negotiate this kind of scene fully. You need to talk to your partner about this kind of play before you get involved with it. You need to see if they are okay with it and even then you should start very slowly.

When we talk about humiliation, we might start with something as simple as calling your partner a little slut while you are having sex, or dirty girl, or that they are a bad boy.

 This is a beginning to see how they react to something that seems fairly tame, but it can be the beginning to much more.

When we are practicing BDSM, we are often playing with power. So, playing around with wrong, and the topics we discuss here, are displays of power. Going against social custom and good taste has a special power to it.

In a vanilla parallel, in our society, the "women love bad boys" phenomenon is debated endlessly. Dr. John Gray, PhD, author of the popular relationship book *Men Are from Mars, Women Are from Venus,* received the following question:

> *"Why is it some of us women are attracted only to the bad boys?"*

The answer Dr. Gray gave was:

> *"What makes any man charismatic is his ability to exude self-confidence. To make a relationship work, a man must not only be confident and assertive, but consider it an empathetic to his partner's needs. A bad boy has the former traits without the latter. While this creates an initial magnetism that is exciting at first, in the long run, his partner will figure out that she deserves better and move on."*

This is a very interesting observation and really shows how BDSM could fit into this equation. We are *playing* around with being the "bad boys and girls". Only playing. Our partner never has to worry about deserving better and moving on. We can play around with that part of the dynamic that is so exciting and magnified.

Basically, a top or a dominant can be a bad boy or a bad girl and give a partner the excitement that they crave, and because we are playing in a consensual safe spaces after we are done playing, we go right back to having an equal relationship with the respect and dignity that all partners deserve from each other.

Wrong is wrong, and as safe, sane and consensual intelligent people, we know that. So, that's what makes it fun. We get to play around with power. We unleash the demon within and play around with taboo subjects all the name of sexual and mental excitement.

It is important to point out that for most of us, playing around with wrong would not work if our partners did not love it deep down inside. This does not work without a connection.

Truth be told, the most exciting thing for many reaction junkies is making their partner understand that the horrible things that I am saying to them are exactly what they want me to do. Making someone face these feelings of excitement can be the most fun of all. Playing with shame is very powerful.

We have been taught since we were a little boy or girl not to shame ourselves. We are taught that our sense of right and wrong and our word is all that we have. So, if you can make your partner admit that they'd sell out the world just for you to let them have an orgasm, that can be a lot of fun and very, very exciting.

Playing around with someone when they are close to orgasm can be terrible fun. It can be seriously shocking what someone will say or do when they are close to orgasm. There is something extremely exciting about making someone face the fact that we are all just animals with animalistic needs, and that when someone is approaching an orgasm, all social conventions usually go out the window in the name of a good orgasm.

Doing this sort of play takes an amazing amount of trust. It is a real turn on to be trusted to that degree and then play with this power.

Your partner knows that you know that they are mortified, and that you could tell someone or next time you are playing, remind her of the terrible things they said and did the last time you played. Your partner needs to be able to trust you with this information, that you won't actually tell anyone, but just that hint that you might is enough to be very exciting

Playing with sensitive personal subjects evokes intense reactions. The more personal, the more sensitive. Remember that when you do this kind of play, you are taking someone on a journey, and it is important that you bring them back to the start of that journey and put them back together at the end.

Be ready to reassure someone it's normal to say and do just about anything to achieve an orgasm. It does not make them a bad person that hearing these dirty thoughts made them have a harder orgasm than they ever had before. Make sure you are giving someone the proper aftercare, as this is the kind of subject where aftercare is often needed days into the future. You want to check in with your partner at least the next day and make sure they feel okay about themselves after doing something as intense as we are discussing.

Rituals and protocols

Rituals and protocols are also mental aspects of the scene which are more corrective or instructional.

As far as rituals go, many bottoms and submissives welcome various different training protocols, which remind them of their submission. For example, every time your playtime starts, you may request that your partner kneels down and bows their head.

This is a very intense way to get your partner in the right headspace or mood for what is about to happen. If this is done every single time as a ritual, every time your partner goes into the playroom or if you decide to begin a playtime, they will naturally go to their position and start to think about what's about to come. Rituals can be very fulfilling to human beings. We do them all the time in the vanilla world.

Creating rituals for your partner can be as simple as getting your coffee every morning. And here is where certain things can spill over from playtime and be carefully added into the vanilla world if that works for you both.

As another example, to show their submission, your partner may greet you when you come home in a certain way or bring you your newspaper once you've settled into your favorite chair.

Little things that can be done just to remind that person that they are your submissive. Again, this is not something that needs to be done, but is a fun model that you may choose to use.

Many people will never want to do anything outside of playtime, even outside of the bed itself. That's fine, but for others, this can be very powerful.

Protocols would be the teaching of the actual way that the dominant wants the partner to serve the coffee or the way they wish to greet the partner at the door or what position they will be in when they kneel down on the floor.

Remember, this is a creative process, and there are no rules or right or wrong protocols. The point is for you to have fun creating your own rituals and your own protocols, whichever call out to you.

There are lots of models and lots of different ones that other people use, and I'm sure you can find many of them on the Internet. However, there is no need to feel that you need to use existing rituals and protocols. Make up your own; have a great time.

SAFETY

Safety is a very serious subject in the BDSM world.

While we are having a good time and enjoying ourselves, we are playing around with pointy objects and various different, potentially dangerous situations, so we must be very careful.

I do not think I am overstating anything by saying:

You have your partner's life in your hands when you are participating in BDSM.

Of course, if you are having a little spanking in the bedroom, there is much less, if not zero chance, of someone losing their life. However, as you start playing with more intense situations, you truly do have your partner's life in your hands.

This should be a mantra that you never forget through all your days in the scene. It is easy to become overconfident, and then next thing you know, something terrible can happen.

Am I trying to scare you?

Yes, I am!

It is far more important that you err on the side of caution.

Every dominant has that a-ha moment at some point on their journey. My job is to help you minimize the chance of something truly bad happening when that moment comes, by being aware of the possibilities.

I am going to tell you a story about my a-ha moment, which happened many, many years ago when I first started out in the scene.

Back before the Internet, when dinosaurs roamed the earth and people actually used payphones, there was something we called a BBS. A BBS was where you would dial in to a computer and chat with each other through a very rudimentary black and white, text interface.

I was a member of one of the most popular BDSM BBS' of the late 80's, which was called The English Palace. This was a wonderful group of people who I still to this day am honored to have been associated with. This is where I met my mentors Philip Miller and Molly Devon, who wrote the book *Screw the Roses, Send Me the Thorns*, a book, by the way, that I recommend highly.

One day while typing on the BBS, I started chatting with a friend named sub Leah, who I was pretty good friends with at the time. We often talked and flirted with each other online.

While we were chatting in a public room, a dominant who was very new came in and started talking to us. Back in those days, sometimes people would actually type out a play scenario while they were chatting, which was called "hot chat", and this new dominant started talking and hot chatting with Leah.

I could tell that he was very new by some of the things he was saying. First off, he was very belligerent and trying to act like what he *thought* a dominant should act like, and he was pretty disrespectful in general. For whatever reason, sub Leah, who was a strong and powerful women, was putting up with this dominant's silly attitude. As he started hot chatting with Leah, he started talking about using a crop on her. He talked about hitting her on the butt, hitting her on the thigh, and he talked about going down the thigh and hitting her down her leg, on the knee, and on the shin.

Leah immediately typed "safeword, release me" and promptly left the chat room. I chuckled to myself, watching sub Leah schooling this new dominant. He had broken a major rule, by talking about hitting Leah somewhere that was not safe to hit (The knee and shin have bone directly underneath and are not good areas to hit. Note: more on this below).

I then explained this to the new dominant that next time, being a little more humble might make him more desirable to other subs, and that he should not hit somebody over bone that it is not a good place to hit. The gentleman grumbled a few words of thanks and left.

I then private messaged Leah and very proudly explained to her how I had set this young man straight. Leah then said to me:

> *"I am not mad at him…*
>
> *I am mad at you."*

I could not believe what I was hearing. Mad at me? What did I do? And then Leah gave me some of the best advice that I have ever gotten, and I remember it as if it was yesterday.

She said, "You and I were together in that room and we were playing. This man came in and you let him play with me. When you let him play with me, he then hurt me. And that is your fault. You were responsible for me."

I could not believe what I was hearing. I tried to explain how this was "on the BBS" and was just silly fun," that "I would never have let that happen in real life."

"I would have watched over you and not allowed anyone to hurt you in real life," I assured.

Leah countered with:

"Are you sure?"

"What if we had been in a public place and there had been a lot of people around, and someone very well-known in the scene came up to you and said, 'Can I play with your partner? Would you have been intimidated into letting him play with me? Even though you didn't know them personally and couldn't vouch for them?"

At that moment, my blood ran cold as even though I hoped that I would never have done what she suggested, being that I was fairly new myself, I realized that it could have been possible. Leah was teaching me a fabulous lesson, and I thank her for it to this day.

Your submissive's life is in your hands. Whether you are playing privately in the bedroom at home, or out in public with other

people, at no point can you ever allow yourself to let your guard down and take things lightly.

When someone is in restraint or you are using a potentially dangerous toy or even just something that could be emotionally damaging to your partner, you need to always be on your highest alert to play as safely as you possibly can.

Now, let's cut to 20 something years later with me playing with one of my partners out at a club. We were playing in a booth in a club in NYC at a party called "Suspension". Now, my partner enjoys being frightened by having a knife involved in our scenes and I had one out and was dragging it across her chest.

This was not for cutting or doing any kind of advanced play, but merely a way to frighten the person. As we sat in that booth, I menaced her with the knife and she was very excited and squirmed around while I had her under control with a handful of hair in my other hand. This was very exciting for my partner, and she was having a great time.

I, then, for one second lost my concentration and looked away at something that was happening over to my left. At that exact moment, my partner suddenly moved to one side and missed impaling her eye on the knife by about an inch.

Had she poked herself with the knife, would it have been my fault? I say yes. I say that it is my responsibility to be aware, to not allow any distractions to keep me from focusing on the most important thing, which is my partner in front of me.

At that moment, I safeworded to myself and stopped the scene. I was shaken and disappointed in myself. After all my experience, after all my teaching novices for years and years how to be safe, I almost permanently injured one of my partners.

Now, you may think I am being too hard on myself, that accidents can happen. And you are right, accidents can happen. However, I could have been doing more to protect my partner, and:

I can never allow myself to think that mostly paying attention is good enough.

If I had been 100 percent focused on the situation and she had accidently gotten hurt, I could have forgiven myself, but in this situation, I would not have been able to.

We are not perfect, mistakes will happen. You may lose concentration sometimes, it is almost inevitable, but if these stories do one thing for you, I hope that they will sit in the back of your brain, and when you do lose concentration at some point, you will remember my words and snap back to being fully present and in the moment with your partner, for this is the only way you should be when you are participating in BDSM activities.

When you are new and you are playing in public or with other people, it is very difficult not to want to show off a bit. We are having a lot of fun and camaraderie is a big part of public play. However, we must keep our head about us and remember that when we are in the midst of noise and large crowds and many distractions:

Nothing matters except for your partner. No person, no thing, no sound, no action.

As you go through your journey, there are certainly times and places where you are more at risk than others. If you are going to be playing at home only with your steady partner, and you know them very well, you certainly will be in the safest environment you could hope for. But, you still need to always be vigilant as you never know what could happen or what could go wrong. Regardless of the venue, NEVER let your guard down,

Your partner deserves your best every time.

As we venture out into the world and play with new partners or go online and meet people in the scene, there are additional things to consider.

When going online and using websites, such as FetLife.com, which we have recommend highly, there are a few good things that you should do to protect yourself.

I suggest that you use an alias. You should not use your real name, at least in the beginning, for safety sake. You should also consider whether you want to show pictures of yourself fully. Some people take pictures where they do not show the face, and that certainly helps.

The reason you are doing this is not just because you may be worried of being outed and people finding out that you are interested in this, but, also, it is a safety measure for unsavory types who might think it's acceptable to show up on your doorstep one day.

It is a very good idea to keep a certain amount of anonymity when you are getting involved in the scene. If you do decide that you want to meet or play with somebody who you do not know, you should be extra careful. That does not mean that the person isn't someone you like or admire or think is a good person, it just means that you don't know them well enough to trust them with your life, yet.

You never want to be alone with somebody who you do not have a long history or relationship with without taking some precautions. One of those precautions is to actually play in public or play around other people.

Now that, of course, might not work for those of you who are interested in having a monogamous partner and playing one-on-one in your home or bedroom, and that is fine. We will discuss some ways to protect yourself there in a minute.

However, if you do meet people outside of your home, playing in a small group or having someone nearby is extremely advantageous as they would be there to help if anything happened where your limits were being disregarded or you are injured in some way.

If you ever have the opportunity to play in a public play space, not only can that be quite exciting, but that may be the very safest place of all as there are many, many people there who are experienced and they will come running should you scream "red" or "safeword".

But to those of you who would never venture out or more than likely won't be doing that too often, you may very well have a situation where you are going to play with somebody new and play with them privately. There are several things you can do to be as safe as possible in this situation.

One would be to be to play in your home and have somebody in the house. This obviously is not going to work out if no one knows about your proclivity or you do not feel comfortable having somebody nearby. But if you do, having somebody watching TV in the living room while you are having a great time in the bedroom is a great way for you to stay safe.

Another thing that we do is what's called a safe call. This can be very effective and all you have to do to set one up is tell a friend that:

You will be calling them at a certain time. If you do not call by that time, they should call you. If you do not answer, they should call the police.

This is not something to be taken lightly as you are asking a friend to call the police to come save you and you may just have lost track of time. That can certainly result in an embarrassing situation. But I will take embarrassment every time over injury or something worse.

Also, you need to make sure that the person you are playing with knows that you have set up the safe call. This creates a deterrent. If for some reason, the person you are playing with was thinking about crossing your limits, they certainly may think about it twice if they know that the police will be called if you cannot respond at a certain time.

Another thing that is very important is to get references. In today's day and age of emails and the

Internet, it is fairly easy for you to check up on somebody. If you meet somebody on a website like FetLife.com, you can ask them for references of other people on FetLife.com that can vouch for them. Also, asking for their vanilla Facebook webpage can be a good idea as well, giving you more information. If someone won't give you their vanilla Facebook, this doesn't mean they are necessarily dangerous. They may be nervous that YOU are a lunatic and going to hurt them somehow as well.

While these are not fool proof methods, they certainly can set up dummy accounts as references and have friends cover for them, you can hopefully have them give you enough information that you feel comfortable being alone with them.

Be very wary of anyone who does not cooperate with your attempts to check them out in the kink world. This a normal thing and very common.

If you are going to venture out and find people on FetLife.com or any other public settings, I strongly urge you to make friends within that community over and above potential play partners. There is nothing that will help you more than other people who are in the same situation as you that you can bounce ideas off of and ask for advice.

Even if you plan to never go out in the scene and never ever look for a new partner, it is still a great idea to make friends with other people on a place like FetLife.com so that you can ask questions and get good information. You can never have too many friends, and having different friends with different opinions and different ways of doing things is one of the best ways to grow and learn.

A few safety tips for when you are actually in a scene and you are alone.

Even if you pretend otherwise, never ever leave your bottom in bondage and alone. While it sounds hot:

Going in to make yourself a sandwich while your submissive struggles in her ropes is not safe.

It is easy for you to give the illusion of this by simply blindfolding your partner, opening and closing the door, but not really leaving and just staying still and watching.

Make sure you have water nearby, a warm blanket, and first aid supplies somewhere close by as well.

Here is a good opportunity to talk about what we call aftercare.

Aftercare is simply what happens after the scene is done. This is a very important part of the scene and should not be taken lightly. Everybody has different ways of processing a scene after it is completed.

Some people go into a sort of semi-shock state where they need warm blankets, cuddles and lots of attention. Other people will become very agitated and need to be left alone. This is not a problem. This just how certain people internalize the scene. You should not be offended nor try to change the way they process. If your partner feels better getting away and being in a different place or different room than you, let them go. Let them process and then you can come back together.

Sometimes aftercare can go on for many days, with the partners checking in with each other over that period of time. Remember, this is a contact sport in both a physical and mental way, so sometimes we hit a speed bump that doesn't present itself right away.

You may do a scene that pushes some of your buttons, but not realize it right away. It may take a day or even weeks before your mind processes it. When this kind of situation happens, the bottom needs to check in with their top and let them know of such a situation. Also a good top will check in with their partner after their play time if they think such a situation is possible.

Remember, the top needs aftercare too. Often, the top may feel some guilt or shame about what has happened, and they may need just as much cuddling and affection afterwards so that they do not feel like they are a bad person.

Sometimes, your aftercare models will not line up. When that is the case, you need to communicate with your partner and figure out a way for you to both get what you need. For example, if someone needs to get away from the other person immediately, yet the other partner needs cuddling, perhaps you might agree together to give the first person 10-15 minutes to be alone before they will come back and cuddle and support the other after they have had a few minutes to be on their own.

Aftercare is a time to reconnect with your partner. This is a great time to just cuddle and be together. After a bit, sometimes it can be a great time to talk about the scene while it is fresh in both your minds, and talk about what was good, what was not so good, what was great, and what was bad.

For some people, this won't be something they like to do, since verbal communication can take them out of their headspace.

Other Safewords

When playing, regardless of where and when, remember, you must keep your scene consensual. So if you are using a gag or playing very loud music or doing something where, for some other reason, a simple safeword will not do, you need to make sure that you plan appropriately.

When someone is gagged, one of the things that you can do is to tell them that, if they grunt three times, for example, that will be a safeword. If you have someone over your knee and are spanking them, you can tell them to grab your ankle if they want to safeword.

Another thing to do is what we call a drop. That would be to simply put something in the person's hand that they hold onto. If they drop it, they have "safeworded".

It is also good for that object to be something a little bit heavier so that it will be more obvious when it is dropped, a rubber ball versus a silk scarf, for example.

Drinking, Drugs, and Playing

Drinking or doing drugs and playing are definitely frowned upon in the BDSM scene and for good reason.

As we noted before, your life is in someone's hands when you are playing, and you certainly do not want to have your life in the hands of someone who is drunk or high.

Now, some people swear by the fact that they need a glass of wine to relax in order to play. Is a glass of wine too much? Is a little bit of pot smoking too much?

I like to use the driving-the-car analogy. If you want one drink and one drink does not affect you to the point where you cannot drive a car, then I think while it would be better not to have anything at all, that would be a good way to gage whether you are able to participate.

If you are not sober enough to drive, you are not sober enough to play.

This goes for both the top and the bottom. Sometimes, people think it does not matter if the bottom is high or drunk, but that is absolutely not so. When you are in an altered state of consciousness, you are not going to be aware of your levels of pain. You will not be able to hold up your end of the consensual bargain. Negotiating while drunk or high is also not a good idea as you may consent to things you would not normally consent to when in an unaltered state of consciousness.

Altered States, a different kind of high

When a bottom plays, they may sometimes experience an altered state of mind that is referred to as subspace or flying. This is usually a pleasant feeling where you feel floaty, lightheaded or otherwise different from your natural state of mind.

Sub Space is a kind of euphoria and natural high that you are getting from all the chemicals that your body is producing during both physical and mental play.

There is also a similar state called top space or dom space that the top can sometimes get into. Although this state of mind can be very similar to what a bottom experiences, it is often more of a hyper awareness or almost hypnotic state.

Conversely, much like a sugar crash, there is both top drop and sub drop that can effect someone after they are finished playing or at the end of a very long play session.

This can be both mental and physical. Indeed, sometimes the body is having an actual sugar drop after heavy physical activity, but also the body can go into a type of shock after a scene.

Also on the mental side regret, shame and various negative feelings can creep in at the end of a scene. During the scene, many different chemicals are coursing through your body; once they wear off, there is a physical change that can affect your mental state deeply.

Where to Hit

One of the biggest questions that I get is "where it is safe to hit people on their bodies?" I am going to tell you a secret. Believe it or not, there have been very few studies done on BDSM. So, unfortunately, we are pretty much on our own listening to various informed sources within our community.

That said, we've come up with a pretty good standard as to where are the safer places to hit. Remember, this is a contact sport. There is no 100-percent-safe anything. People will ask me, "if I hit somebody near the heart, can I stop their heart?" Yes, you can. Will you *probably* stop the heart? No.

We always hear about some regrettable situation in which someone is killed playing a sport, but there are certainly hundreds of thousands of other people who are not killed when the same exact thing happens. If you are looking for 100 percent safety, you should not play with corporal punishment or any kind of physical play.

This all said, let's move on to where are the safest places to hit and the places to avoid.

In general, you should look for places thickly covered in fat and muscle. Fat and muscle are perfect because they can absorb the blow and protect the organs underneath. Although hitting fatty or muscular areas may leave marks, it is likely there will be little or no damage to a bone, nerve or organ. You do not want to hit places on the body where there are bones very close to surface of the skin, where many, many nerves come together, or where organs are very close to where you are hitting.

You are going to find that there are some places that people generally feel are good to hit that still have nerves or bones or organs close by. The idea is not to make yourself crazy with this. This is not an exact science. The idea is for you to learn the saf-ER spots so you can stay in those areas.

When I am watching people play at events, occasionally, I see somebody who is lightly touching somebody on their kidney area or other such *warning area* and someone nearby will grumble, "hey, that guy is hitting his kidneys. That is wrong."

On one hand I'm glad that the person is aware of the bad areas to hit, but I'm also unnerved by the lack of common sense the person is showing. If I run my fingers up and down someone's body and run them over somebody's kidneys, I am not going to hurt them. As a matter of fact, it is going to feel very nice.

Similarly, if you hit someone super lightly on a bad spot, that does not mean that you are injuring them. Just refrain from hitting them hard in the same area.

B*ad spots* to hit are the bones, nerves and organs. Some boney places where you'd want to stay away from are: your shins, your knee, your elbows, the tops of your feet. Any place where you know there are bones sitting right there that you can almost see, obviously, your ribs and places like that, are all places that are not as good to hit.

With nerves, the spine, insides of the wrist, around the neck, the tops of the shoulders, behind the knees are all places where many nerves can be found.

As far as organs go, probably the most commonly talked about would be the kidneys, which are on the lower left and right walls of the back. Your kidneys are very, very close to the surface, and you would not want to repeatedly hit in that spot.

The butt is the best place to hit on the body. It is the most well-muscled and fat-covered place on the body. When you are starting out in the scene, hitting the butt is your very best spot to start with. Not the top of the butt, but from the middle of the butt down. Once you are getting higher up on the butt, you have the coccyx bone very close, and you want to stay away from that.

So from mid-butt down is a perfect place to hit. And we have what is called the sweet spot, which is where people's legs meet their butts. This is a spot that some people feel is the best spot to hit, other people think it is the worst. You will have to communicate with you partner and see. But your butt, the sweet spot, and then the thighs, front and back, are all well-muscled, fatty places that you can hit.

Next is the upper back. There are spots on the back that are very well-muscled towards the inside middle part of the back. You can feel with your fingers where the muscle is, but the entire back of the area that covers the top third of your back is a good place to hit with a flogger or other such toy. Stay away from the very top of the back/shoulders/neck area. These are all places you do not want to hit.

The chest area, (not the breasts guys, that's different, see comments below) can be a bit difficult to get to with certain toys, but is an excellent place to hit. It is well muscled and can take hard play. Just make sure the person you are playing with has their chin up and head back.

You will often see people using a flogger and crossing over the entire back, and I am often asked, "isn't that bad because it covers the spine?" And the spine certainly has bones and nerves in it. The answer is when throwing a whip, whether it is a flogger or a single-tail whip, what is going fast are the tips. When you are using a flogger across the back, make sure to aim the tip to the right or left of the spine. You will find that when you are crossing over the spine, the middle of the flogger is just giving a thuddy feel to the rest of the back.

That said, if you have a partner whose spine is extremely close to the surface, it could protrude from the back, so it is probably less of a good idea to hit across the back.

Again, communication. Talk to your partner. Does that hurt a lot in a bad way when I do that? Just ask.

Other okay places to hit are the calves. The calves are very, very well-muscled, just maybe not quite as pleasurable to feel and also the sides of the upper arms have been the spot teenage boys have delighted in punching each other since the dawn of time.

Places to hit lightly, The bottoms of the feet are tricky, many people like what is called bastinado. Bastinado is the hitting of the bottoms of the feet. While you should be careful because there are many bones in the feet, the bottom is much better to hit than the top.

Also be careful with the genitals and inner thighs. Inner thighs have a lot of nerves, so be careful, but they can be great places to hit. Also, the genitals can be hit lightly, but, obviously, be very careful there. The penis itself is very resilient and can take a lot. The testicles, however, are a completely different spot and should be avoided. Not only can the pain be unbearable, this is not a place you want to damage. A woman's private parts can be extremely sensitive, however, they can usually take quite a bit of intensity if you both enjoy this.

The stomach can be hit, but it would be best if the person was tensed up and their muscles were clenched in their stomach. Obviously, the stomach has a whole six pack of abdominal muscles to protect it, but you want to be careful and go lightly.

The breasts can be a fun place to hit, but you have to be very careful. Again, going back to the concept that very few medical studies have been done in the name of BDSM, we do not know how dangerous hitting the breast might be.

Many people are very susceptible to developing cysts or tumors. This is something that you have to negotiate with your partner. I see many people hitting breasts, but that does not make it right. So, make sure you ask your partner if they have a family history of this kind of problem. If so, it's probably not a good idea to do anything but the lightest play on the breasts.

Places that are absolutely bad would be directly on the spine, the lower back, the sides of the hips, the tops of the feet, and the head and neck. As far as the arms go, there are lots of bones in the hands. So other than possibly the bicep and sides of the arms, it's probably best to leave them alone.

Again, remember, if you make a mistake and hit somebody on the kidney or neck or some other bad spot once, it is very doubtful they will have to go to the hospital. You want to use common sense and realize that you will always make a bad hit here and there. These things happen, but the idea is to not repeatedly be hitting a bad spot.

Don't make yourself so crazy about a bad hit someplace that you are afraid you have injured the person severely. Of course, if you hit anything hard enough even once you could do quite a bit of damage, but for just normal play, you do not need to worry so much that it affects your play. Just stay away from the bad spots.

Also, don't be afraid. If you do make a bad hit, simply touch that spot and ask the person if they are okay. There is nothing wrong with checking in and admitting a mistake. As a matter of fact, it builds trust with your partner so they know that you are aware of the mistake and care enough to try and avoid repeating it.

Warming Up

Remember, when you are doing any kind of pain play, warming up is important. The person does not feel things the same when cold as they do once they are warmed up. A person will be able to take a lot more pain if they are warmed up slowly. Also, remember this important tidbit, everybody interprets pain differently. So, when you play with one person, their heavy might be another person's light, and vice versa. Also, people's pain tolerance changes day to day, minute to minute or mindset to mindset, especially females whose bodies change constantly over the course of a month.

As I said in the beginning of this chapter, remember the most important thing is to not get so caught up in your technique or anything else that is going on that you are not paying attention to your partner. Your connection to your partner is more important than anything. You and your partner are one. When you are playing, the only thing you should be paying attention to is each other.

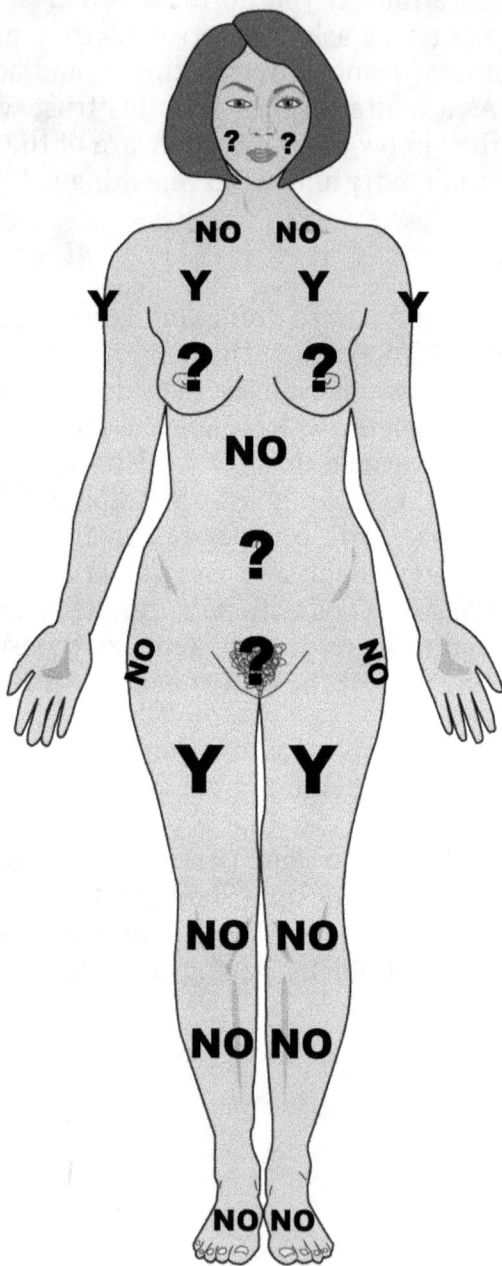

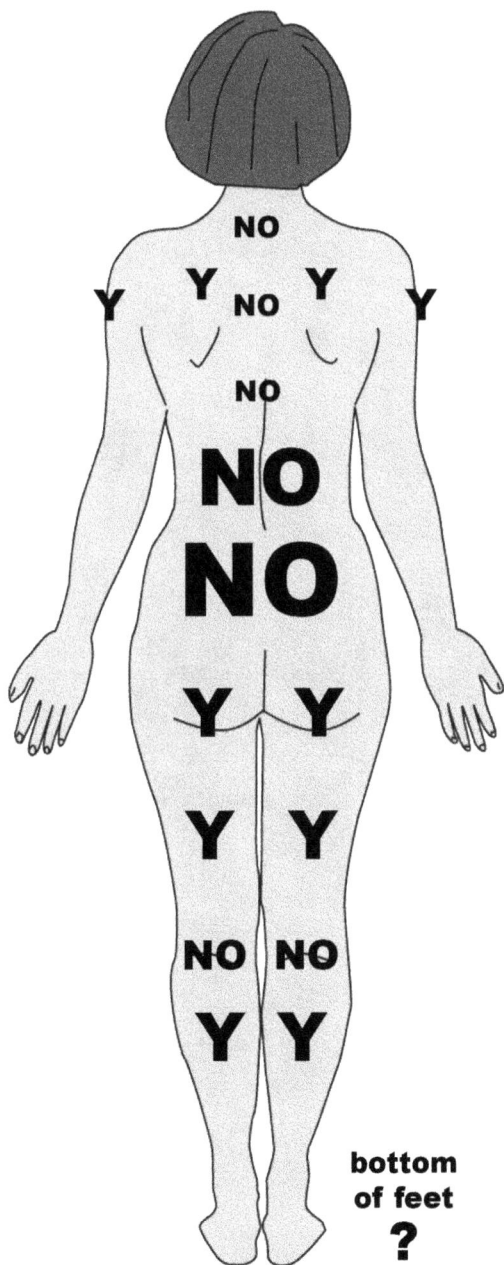

NO

Y NO Y Y

NO

NO

NO
NO

Y Y

Y Y

NO NO

Y Y

bottom
of feet
?

IN CONCLUSION

I hope you have enjoyed this overview of beginning BDSM. I've dedicated a big part of my life to helping people play safely, sanely, and consensually in our scene, and my goal was to put together an easy read, that would give you a feel for what is out there.

Please check out my reading list below for more great books on BDSM and alternative sexuality.

And remember:

When you stop growing, you start dying...

So let go of your fears,

Seek truth and

Find your integrity

READING LIST

There are many other wonderful books that I am fond of and recommend for pleasure reading and education. I've included some here, but you can also visit my website at *www.alternativelifecoach.com/readinglist* for links to all of them.

My good friend Laura Antoniou is a legend in the realm of BDSM fiction. Her Marketplace series is a classic that you'll find in just about every serious player's bookshelf.

- *The Marketplace*

- *The Slave* (Marketplace book #2)

- *The Trainer* (Marketplace book #3

Anne Rice, writing under the pen names of A. N. Roquelaure and Anne Rampling, may truly be the mother of the modern erotic novel. These were the first fantasy BDSM books I ever read, so they have a special place in my heart. The Beauty trilogy and *Exit to Eden* are favorites of mine.

- *The Claiming of Sleeping Beauty*

- *Beauty's Punishment* (Sleeping Beauty book #2)

- *Beauty's Release* (Sleeping Beauty book #3)

- *Exit to Eden*

Cecilia Tan and all our friends at Circlet Press have some of the best erotic fiction around. Check out any books put out by them.

Susan Wright is the founder of the National Coalition of Sexual Freedom. For that reason alone you should buy her books! She is a well known professional writer of many a genre, including 9 Star Trek novels. But for this list, you'll be more interested in her awesome, kinky fantasy books. Her classic *Slave Trade* has just been re-released.

Here are my favorite BDSM educational books:

Screw the Roses, Send Me the Thorns: The Romance and Sexual Sorcery of Sadomasochism – This book is near and dear to my heart as it was written by my first mentors, the now deceased Philip Miller and Molly Devon. This book is written about the NJ BDSM community in the late 80's and is a classic.

The Ethical Slut: A Practical Guide to Polyamory, Open Relationships & Other Adventures – The single most influential book on Polyamory or as we in the scene like to say "ethical non-monogamy", which is a phrase that I stole from this book. If you are interested in this type of relationship, you *need* this book.

The Loving Dominant – This classic is written by my old friend John Warren. A great read.

Books by Tristan Taormino – I love, love, love me some Tristan T! She has written a TON of great books

Different Loving: The World of Sexual Dominance and Submission – A true classic by Gloria Brame.

Learning the Ropes: A Basic Guide to Safe and Fun S/M Lovemaking – Written by Race Bannon, founder of Kink Aware Professionals and a wonderful man I admire greatly.

SM 101: A Realistic Introduction – This is another classic written by Jay Wiseman.

Topping and Bottoming Books - From the people that brought you *The Ethical Slut*.

BDSM The Naked Truth – Our friend Dr. Charley's latest book.

The Toybag Guide Series – I have not read all of the books in this series, but some of my favorite people in the scene have written these, like Lolita Wolf, Lee Harrington, Mollena Williams, Midori, John Warren and more.

Leatherman's Handbook II – This classic by Larry Townsend is no longer in print, but there are a few used copies that you can pick up on Amazon. This is a great book for everyone, but gives the gay male dominant perspective.

And if you are interested in more of an anthropological view, here are three books I LOVE.

Sex at Dawn: How We Mate, Why We Stray, and What It Means for Modern Relationships – This book by Christopher Ryan and Cacilda Jetha is one of the most inspiring and important things I've ever read. See a short blog post on it here.

Playing on the Edge: Sadomasochism, Risk, and Intimacy – My dear friend Dr. Staci Newmahr, has written an absolutely amazing book, that is as ruthlessly honest as it is thought provoking. A sociologist and ethnographer, she participated in the NYC BDSM scene for several years to give a firsthand account of what she experienced. Written as academic book, this is still required reading for those that want an inside look at the NYC BDSM scene in the late 2000's

Leatherfolk: Radical Sex, People, Politics, and Practice – One of my favorite books! If you are interested in leather history and human sexuality, this is a classic must-read. *Leatherfolk* is both a historical witness and provocative treatise regarding the leather subculture from the 1940's onward.

Your favorite fiction

These books were suggested by my followers on social media and at my website.

- **Books by Charise Sinclair** – Many suggest this author.

- **Mercy, Comfort Object and Books by Annabel Joseph**

- **Learning to Drown and Books by Sommer Marsden**

- *Coming to Power*, *Macho Sluts* **and books by Patrick Califia** – Patrick Califia's writing and activism have revolutionized queer sex.

- **Books by Anneke Jacobs**

- *Master/slave Relations* **and Many Books by Robert J. Rubel**

- **The Safeword Series and Books by Candace Blevins**

- **The Order of Solace Series and Books by Megan Hart**

- *Nature of Desire* **and The Boardroom Series and Books by Joey W. Hill**

- *Tied to Passion* **and Books by Amber Rose Thompson** – BDSM erotica with a flair for the romantic and sometimes the added spice of the paranormal.

- *Bared to You* **and Books by Sylvia Day**

- **Books by Sadey Quinn**

- *Dommemoir* **and many books by I.G. Frederick**

- *Gabriel's Inferno* **by Sylvain Reyard -Many suggest, but no BDSM**

- **The Sinners on Tour Series and Books by Olivia Cunning**

- ***The Reluctant Dom, Domme by Default, Love Slave for Two*, and Books by Tymber Dalton** – *The Reluctant Dom* is finally available again on Amazon.

- ***Kushiel's Dart* and Books by Jacqueline Carey**

- ***The Story of O* by Pauline Reqge**

- **The Sweet Series by Maya Bank's** – Several suggest this author.

- ***Carrie's Story* and *Safe Word*, Books by Molly Weatherfield aka: Pam Rosenthal**

- ***Beautiful Disaster* and Books by Jamie McGuire**

- ***Thoughtless* and *Effortless* by S.C. Stephens**

- ***100 Strokes of the Brush Before Bed* by Melissa P.**

- ***Hearts in Darkness* by Laura Kaye**

- ***Becoming Sage, Saving Sunni* and Books by Kasi Alexander**

- **Books by Tammy Jo Eckhart** – Interesting female dominant, vampires and more.

- ***The Dark Garden, The Darker Side of Pleasure* and books by Eden Bradley**

- *Masters at Arms* and The Rescue Me Series, and Books by Kallypso Masters

- *The Marriage Bargain* and Books by Jennifer Probst

- *Damaged Goods* and Books by Lauren Gallagher

- The Rendezvous Series by Victoria Blisse

- *Entertainment for a Master* and Books by John Preston – Great gay male BDSM

- *A Table for Three* by Lainey Reese

- Books by Shakir Rashaan

- *Consensual Sadomasochism : How to Talk About It & Do It Safely* by Sybil Holiday and William A. Henkin

- *Crow's Row* by Julie Hockley

- *Once Upon a Temptation* by Kaye P. Hallows

- *Protégée* and Books by Dakota Lynn

- Books by Lora Leigh

- *Corporal in Charge of Taking Care of Captain O'Malley* by Jack Fritscher

- The Anita Blake and Merry Gentry series by Laurell K. Hamilton

- ***Playing With Pain: Stories from My Life in Leather*** by Hardy Haberman

- ***PA Exposé*** by Kristal Baird

- ***The Puppy Papers: A Woman's Journey into BDSM*** by Puppy Sharon and Steven Toushin

- ***Her Own Serenity*** by Julia Becca

Remember, you can also visit my website at *http://www.alternativelifecoach.com/readinglist* for links to all of these books.

BO'ISMS

"My job in life is to help people lose their fear, seek the truth, and find integrity."

"When You stop growing, you start dying."

"You are exactly where you should be... NOW WHAT?"

"In the absence of truth, a person is sure to beat themselves up for the rest of their life over the silence."

"You have to be willing to lose to gain."

"Shake your life, often and vigorously. Don't let the snowflakes ever hit the bottom of your globe. Life is far too short to settle."

"Nothing creates serenity like integrity."

"Being a coach isn't about being perfect, it's about inspiring people to play big. Having the confidence to face your humanity, and understand that you are not playing big enough if you don't fail sometimes, is a big part of how we do that!"

"Fear, fornication, and food run the world."

"Personal growth and a quest for knowledge and truth is my spirituality."

"W. Axl Rose is secretly the bastard son of Ethel Merman and a Parrot."

ABOUT THE AUTHOR

Bo Blaze is a PCC-certified "alternative" life coach specializing in alternative sexual relationships and non-traditional lifestyles.

Bo is a nationally known expert on kink, lifestyle BDSM, ethical non-monogamy (polyamory), the fetish world and LGBT issues. He has taught and lectured all over the country at hundreds of universities, conferences and various alternative events.

Bo is the winner of the 2011 Pantheon of Leather President's Award and has helped thousands learn to practice safe, sane and consensual BDSM over the last 10 years as the novice group facilitator and board member emeritus for The Eulenspiegel Society (TES), the oldest and largest BDSM support and education group in the country.

Bo is also the creator and host of the popular online video show, "50 Shades of Curious News"

For more information please visit
www.AlternativeLifeCoach.com
and
www.50ShadesOfCurious.com

INDEX

"24/7", 69 - 71, 74, 76,
   89 -91

A Scene, 15

abuse, 9, 11, 12, 49, 50,
   57, 87, 88, 140

Aftercare, 17, 164, 165

BDSM, iii, 7 - 19, 23, 31,
   34, 41, 47, 49, 53 - 58,
   60 - 70, 72, 75, 76, 80,
   82, 83 - 85, 93 - 96,
   98, 100, 102, 103,
   106, 108, 113, 116,
   133, 134, 139 - 144,
   147, 148, 153, 154,
   158, 166, 168, 172, 177
   - 185, 188

biting, 105

blindfold, 28, 119, 122

bondage, 122 - 124, 163

Bottom, 15, 16

bratting, 109, 110

breath play, 132

bruises, 114

caning, 126

choking, 132

clothespins, 125

collar, 92, 95, 96

Collaring, 69, 70

communication, 10, 23,
   25, 27, 30, 34, 43, 44,
   53, 56, 66, 68, 105,
   116, 134, 138, 142,
   145, 171

Confidence, 98, 99

consensual, 7, 9, 10 - 12,
   15, 21, 22, 49 - 51, 53,
   57, 63, 74, 87, 91, 105,
   122, 131, 132, 136,
   145, 148, 165, 167, 188

Consensual non-
   consent, 131

consent, 11, 12, 16, 31,
   46, 48, 49, 53, 58, 83,
   85, 106, 131, 132, 136,
   137

contact sport, 54, 107, 164, 168

contract, 47, 48, 92, 95

Conversion, 19

corporal, 54, 109, 168

crop, 118, 120, 155

crying, 112, 115, 116

daddy, 18, 63, 64, 75, 80, 93, 136

Defining and Reinventing Yourself, 98

dirty thoughts, 19, 20, 22, 150

discipline, 14, 109

dom space, 167

dominant, 9, 12, 15, 16, 27, 31, 34,56, 61, 62, 64, 65, 67, 71 - 74, 77, 80, 83 - 87, 89, 90, 92 - 94, 96 - 101, 102, 105, 106, 110 - 112, 115, 116, 140, 141, 148, 151, 154, 155, 180, 181, 184

Drinking, 166

drugs, 58, 166

Dungeon, 15

Edge Play, 17, 145

English Palace, 154

Face slapping, 107, 130

fantasy, 21, 22, 25, 32, 33, 89, 104, 136, 137, 138, 178, 179

fear, 9, 20, 21, 24, 29, 41, 77, 78, 81, 130, 186

Fetish, 4, 7, 18, 28, 32, 33, 41,43, 86, 143, 144, 188

Fetlife.com, 17 - 19, 102, 103, 159, 162

Fifty Shades of Grey, 8, 10, 19, 52, 70, 89

Flogging, 3, 36, 37, 127

flying, 167

Gags, 37, 122

guilt, 21, 143, 145, 147, 164

Head Space, 15, 52, 59, 92, 106, 141, 150, 165

homework, 41 - 43, 138, 145

honorifics, 98

humble, 101, 155

humiliation, 28, 31, 141, 142, 145, 147

identify, 14, 16, 31, 63, 67, 80, 82, 84, 87, 93 - 95

inner demon, 103, 105

integrity, 14, 55 - 59, 66, 72, 73, 76 - 78, 99, 139, 140, 177, 178, 186

kinky, 3, 4, 8 - 11, 13, 14, 16, 19, 23 - 25, 27, 29, 30, 34, 55, 71, 73, 77, 83, 86, 100, 102, 144, 179

knives, 130

Limits, 16, 41

Local groups, 18

Master, i, 5, 15, 42, 92, 96, 182, 184

Mental Concerns, 41

Mistress, 15, 92

monogamous, 62, 66, 67, 68, 86, 102, 160

Negotiating, 43, 167

Negotiation, 17, 30

Negotiation Form, 34

negotiation forms, 29, 134, 137, 142, 145

Newbie, 16

Novice, 7, 16

outed, 159

ownership, 69, 70

paddle, 120, 121, 127

pain, 15, 53, 56, 61 - 65, 68, 86, 87, 94, 108 - 112, 114 - 117, 127, 136, 166, 172, 173

Physical Concerns, 41

Play Space, 15

Playing, 15, 33, 74, 142, 143, 146, 149, 150, 166, 181, 185

polyamorous, 16, 57, 62, 63, 66 - 69, 77

polyamory, 7, 16, 66, 68, 82, 179, 188

Power Exchange, 15

Power neutral, 16, 67

primal feelings, 105

Protocols, 151

punishment, 54, 64, 65, 109, 111, 168

RACK, 55

reaction junkies, 112, 143, 144, 149

Relentless pursuit of information, 27

Risk Aware Consensual Kink, 55

role play, 46, 49, 50, 62, 64, 76, 93, 108, 134 - 136, 143

roleplaying, 60, 61, 108, 110, 111, 118

romance, 7 - 10, 60, 61, 62, 72, 179

rope, 122, 123

sadists, 111, 113

safe call, 161

Safe, sane, and consensual, 53

Safety, 123, 153

safety scissors, 123, 124

safeword, 17, 45, 46, 47, 49 - 53, 56, 74, 122, 137, 145, 155, 165, 166

Saran wrap, 124

semantics, 69, 93, 113

service top, 112

shame, 115, 116, 143, 145, 149, 164, 167

slave, 15, 16, 61, 62, 70, 74, 80, 89 - 93, 95 - 98, 178, 179, 183

spanking, 8, 13, 14, 44, 45, 58, 85, 103, 110, 119, 120, 135, 139, 153, 165

SSC, 7, 53, 55

sub drop, 167

Sub Space, 16, 167

submissive, 9, 12, 15, 16, 18, 31, 34, 44, 51, 61, 62, 64, 67, 69, 75, 80, 83, 84, 85 - 87, 89, 91 - 96, 98, 106, 110, 121, 140, 142, 151, 163

Switch, 16

taboo, 17, 22, 31, 116, 136, 142, 143, 145, 146, 149

TES, iii, 7, 19, 80, 82, 98, 188

The Scene, 14

Tickling, 36, 40, 122

Top, 15, 16, 34, 41, 164

top drop, 167

top space, 167

topping from the bottom, 110

trauma, 88, 131

Triangle of Communication, 23

truth, 9, 14, 42, 55, 56, 78, 89, 99, 177, 186, 187

vanilla, 13, 16, 18, 19, 23, 27, 34, 55, 60, 62, 74, 83, 84, 102, 103, 106, 114, 140, 147, 151, 162

verbal communication, 24, 27, 30, 137, 145, 165

whipping, 126, 133

wrong, 8, 13, 20, 21, 25, 26, 50, 54, 55, 69, 80, 85, 86 - 88, 93, 103, 119, 134, 137, 138, 143 - 149, 151, 159, 169, 173